THE LIFE WE GOT

THE LIFE WE GOT

LOSING SIGHT & GAINING VISION

ALISON TAYLOR ▪ NEIL TAYLOR

Printed in the United States of America

First Printing, 2016

ISBN 978-0-9969719-6-6

∾

Photographs by Taylor family
Book and cover design by the Booksmyth,
imprint of Ginger Cat Designs, Shelburne Falls, MA wwwthe-
booksmythpress@gmail.com

For Jim, Jessica and Jackson

The moment in which the mind acknowledges "This isn't what I wanted, but it's what I got" is the point at which suffering disappears. Sadness might remain present, but the mind, having given up the fight for another reality, is free to console, free to support the mind's acceptance of the situation, free to allow space for new possibilities to come into view.

- Silvia Boorstein

CONTENTS

PART THREE: By Grit and by Grace

∿

PREFACE

IN FEBRUARY 2008, MY SON, NEIL, a handsome, athletic twenty-eight year old, underwent surgery for a large, malignant brain tumor and woke to a life of total blindness. Throughout the ensuing challenges of renewing his health, redefining his sense of self, and rebuilding his life, he would say, "I should be writing about this." And I would agree, but the doing of it remained somewhere "out there" like so many dreams and intentions never fulfilled or even begun.

Then one day, a number of years ago now, I visited a friend who casually mentioned that she had been in the presence of a psychic. I cannot remember the details of why; it seemed somewhat out of character for her. But embedded in her own story was a message for me. She said that she had asked about Neil, particularly regarding his health and his future, and that the psychic had said, "I have a good feeling about his life, and I believe that he will write a book."

And that was it. Neil had already expressed a desire—a number of times, in fact —though he didn't really know how or where to start. He may not have truly believed he would or could take on such a project. But, in my mind, a seed lying dormant germinated that day. This was supposed to happen. It was I who had received the message, albeit second hand, and I needed to be part of the endeavor.

Following this unusual incident my awareness began to broaden. Not only did I need to help Neil; I needed to help myself. I, too, needed to write my story of this devastating part of our lives. As a mother I had undergone profound trauma as I witnessed my son dealing with life-threatening cancer and life as a disabled person.

From my personal life as a long-time journal writer and my professional life as a teacher, I believed in the power of writing to make sense of experiences that we are unable to fully process and incorporate into the landscapes of our minds and hearts. I understood that writing can serve as a therapeutic tool to process, to make peace with, and to "own" the unbearable. I looked to this project as a way to put the pieces of me back together.

And so we started. And we started as simply as we could, one step at a time. We chose one scenario—the night Neil called to tell me he had gotten results of an MRI his dad and I didn't know he had had. Neil would write about that night from his perspective, and I would write about it from mine. We would use slightly different fonts to distinguish our individual voices. There would be times in the book in which one of us would have something to relate, and the other would not: Neil could not tell much about his long days of unconsciousness in the hospital; I knew little about his studies at The Carroll Center for the Blind. But we could fold our experiences together to form one story.

This project has been one of the most gratifying yet one of the most difficult experiences of my life. Reliving the events, which, of course, entailed reviving the emotions, was a conscious act fueled by a sense of purpose. There were times I wept, times I laughed out loud, times I sat trying to piece together sequences and details that had faded. Neil and I would confer with each other, then ask others to confirm or contradict the accuracy of our memories. Sometimes it was helpful; other times our "sources" would scratch their heads and wonder, too, how they could have been so seemingly "present" at the time yet fuzzy in the recalling. More than once Neil and I wrote about the same event and, in the sharing, realized that we remembered it somewhat differently. We decided to leave our accounts as we each saw them. Defending our own point of view to each other was less important than sharing our story.

And then there was the writing itself, at times frustratingly, painfully laborious. But it taught me so much. I had to learn to sit and sift, sit and receive, sit and be patient, sit and have faith—like life, itself. And like life, itself, there were unexpected surprises. There were times when the writing and I shifted places. It took over and swept me along with it. On those rare and special days there were no eddies to divert me, no snags to slow my momentum, just a certain "knowing" and rightness to the words that emerged. They were there and I was the channel.

When I started this project, I did not know if it would ever truly become a book. My deepest gratitude goes to my writing partner, Sandra Boston, who met with me every month for two years as we shared excerpts from each other's memoirs. She taught me a great deal about the craft of writing, and one afternoon she said, "You have come this far. You will have to finish this project." And once again, that was that. I knew that I would. It became real to me. This book never would have been born had it not been for a terrible turn of events in our lives. It is a story of suffering and survival. And, for me, it now stands as an offering.

Like everyone who has ever met him, Neil's courage and resolve to forge a happy, meaningful life have affected me deeply by revealing the resilience we humans possess to adapt, to adjust, to persevere. Neil—you have given me many gifts. Two of the most precious are these: you made me a mother, and you made me a writer. Both were dreams I nurtured from a young age. This joint undertaking was long and challenging. We needed to take many breaks. What never stalled, however, was our devotion to each other and our willingness to start over as many times as it took.

Until the end of my days, I will feel blessed to be part of "Team Taylor." To my children, Jessica and Jackson, I couldn't be more proud of the people you are—full of love, courage, and wisdom. And to Jim, whom I recognized as my life's partner when we were oh so young, gratitude beyond words for your ability, your willingness, day after day, again and again, to guide me into the light when I couldn't find it myself.

~ Alison Taylor
Brattleboro, Vermont
April 2016

PREFACE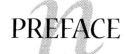

EIGHT YEARS AGO, IF THE PROSPECT of writing a memoir at the age of thirty-six had crossed my mind, I would have dismissed it with a laugh. I would have argued that thirty-six is too tender an age to have gathered enough material, enough life experience, to be ready to share much of substance. I would have assumed that I, like most of my contemporaries, would still be a novice at the hard game of living— a spring chicken in the proverbial coop of life.

But I can't shake the feeling that I have lived nearly a lifetime in the past eight years. Having lost nearly everything that I took for granted—that the majority of young people can and do and probably should take for granted—well, maybe I've earned a sort of cosmic permission to share the story of my life so far.

Like many others who have taken on memoir writing, mine is a story of loss and the long process of facing the facts and mustering the will to enter an unfamiliar existence—an existence I never could have imagined inhabiting. At the same time, my story is unique, as they all are. For me, the facts are these: at the age of twenty-eight I was diagnosed with a large malignant brain tumor and catapulted overnight into total blindness.

In sharing my journey my hope is that someone out there

is helped and sustained in dealing with his or her own life challenge. That possibility brings me happiness. But in all honesty, I took on this project for my own behalf. I needed to face the endless, haphazard swirl my thoughts and feelings had created in my head. To sit alone with the unbearable experiences I'd lived through, to watch them parade in technicolor before me, waiting to be captured and relived, has been a psychological marathon. At the same time, confronting the fragments of my nightmare face to face, with no safety net to catch me if I lost my balance, no pharmaceuticals to ease the pain, has been cathartic and a powerful form of self-therapy. I became aware, as I began writing, that I was embarking on a long struggle to find myself, to become whole. To do this, I had to look a second time at the events I'd lived through. I had to evaluate them for what they were and what they were worth in the remaking of myself.

I am indebted to my parents, my older sister, and my twin brother for their unwavering commitment to stand by my side throughout this rugged journey. And I dedicate my portion of this memoir to my mother Alison. Without her spurring me on with the heartfelt conviction that this story should be out in the world, it never would have been. So many times I'd abandon the project for days or weeks at a time. It was hard enough living the life I'd gotten when I'd had no choice. The pain of reliving it over again, casting light on all the details, and ruminating on the original suffering was a choice and one I could not always stick with. So, while I never wanted to, and never did call it quits, I needed my routine "breaks."

I am convinced that without my mother keeping me on track, my writing would be lost on some unidentified file in a long forgotten folder, stashed away on an outdated laptop in a dusty corner of my own attic never to be discovered or shared. But that will not happen. Gratitude beyond words, Mom, for believing in me and for being my partner for the duration. From scratching our heads in confusion over the sequence of events we were sorting through, to reeling with disbelief in recalling the grimmest of days, to crying together for our losses and laughing at the inevitable comic moments that even our joint life dished up—you were there for me, and I was there for you. And together we created something we can be proud of.

~ Neil Taylor
Brattleboro, Vermont
April 2016

PART ONE

Life Comes Calling

ONE

READY OR NOT

"1, 2, 3, Red Light!"

~ a schoolyard game

*a*I WAS IN "PLANNING MODE" that late afternoon of January 31, 2008, as I bounced through the circuit of exercise machines at the local gym. My husband had left that morning with his mother and brother for their annual trip to Florida, and I was on my own for five whole days. I was rarely home alone for an extended block of time so this mother and sons vacation had become a special time for me as well. I viewed it as a retreat. Suddenly I was face to face with nobody but me! The gift of a quiet house with no social interaction became an opportunity to take stock of my life and to contemplate my own development. This was the first day of my retreat and here I was, not home from work yet, but already doing something good for myself after a busy day in my first and second grade classroom.

I planned my meals for the next couple of nights as I finished my first round on the machines. The second round brought on an image of myself out on the cross-country ski trails down the road from our house followed by my sitting in meditation in my special chair. My energy soared. The choices were all mine, and I felt confident that I could manage the discipline to turn these visions into reality.

This state of optimism and well-being, fueled in part by the workout I'd just completed, enveloped me for the entire twenty-five-minute drive home. How could I not feel that life was good; I was strong and healthy, had a job and family I loved and, foremost on my gratitude meter, my three children were launched in directions that nurtured them and reflected the unique individuals they were.

I thought back over my adult life. I had experienced such joy in the raising of our three babies. And I had done well with masking the many anxieties that come with parenthood—the sometimes overwhelming feelings of responsibility I'd felt for my children's safety, their self-confidence, their intellectual development, their social skills. I had practiced hard at being the relaxed, laid-back mom I wished I truly was. Never mind that, in truth, I was a consummate worry wort. I had modeled for my children that life is a grand adventure to be lived with trust and exuberance, with an open heart and open mind. If I hadn't exactly tamed, I'd at least formed a respectful truce with my humiliating secret belief that I was not naturally a strong person, not someone well equipped to deal with the really tough stuff of life.

But really, who is ever ready? And how can we truly know who we are and what we are made of until we are called upon to travel an unfamiliar and unwelcome path?

I entered my empty house and glanced at the phone. The message light registered three calls, and I dutifully pressed and waited even before setting my packages down. Procrastination would not undermine the "put together" image I was building of myself. I would deal with first things first. And if there was a message from my close friend Judy, just wanting to touch base and chat, I had all the time in the world.

Message number one was a blank. Second up, my son Neil's voice, half an octave lower than usual, tight and clipped—"Mom, as soon as you get this—call me." That kind of message in that timbre of voice sets off warning gongs in anyone. Neil didn't sound like himself. He was generally cheerful, chatty, even teasing when leaving us messages. I pressed again—his voice again, in the same strained tone—"Mom, call me right away."

I knew immediately, intuitively, that the first, blank message had been him as well, trying to contact me about something urgent, something troubling, something that I didn't want to hear.

My feeling of well being congealed in an instant and was replaced by the kind of fear that alters the body's chemistry like a lethal injection. Something was wrong. My maternal intuition was flashing an internal warning.

My first thought went immediately to Neil's job—his first teaching experience which he had come to love, that he was good at, that was his calling, at long last, after floundering for too long. Was he being fired? Was he being accused of something?

I dialed his cell and he answered on the first ring. "Mom, hi," came his voice, a little breathy, as though he'd been rushing. "Listen, I want you to sit down."

And now, I am in a completely different place—transported already from peace and contentment and "all is right with the world." "Neil," I managed, "what is it? You're scaring me!"

We can protect ourselves from hard rain, from dangerous cold, even from vicious gossip. But we have no power over bad news. It is the uncontrollable flood, the avalanche, the tsunami. "Mom," came his trembling voice—"I have a brain tumor."

Why is it that our first response to a message like this is always "WHAT?" like our hearing has suddenly deteriorated or the static of a bad connection has made every second word unintelligible. I know there is a nanosecond between the circuit from ear to brain, but perhaps devastating news, the kind that will change life forever, gets stuck en route because of its toxic charge.

Or maybe that pathetic response of "WHAT?" is our feeble attempt at protection. If we say it, somehow we can start again, and maybe the message will be different and the bearer of bad news will realize that the joke was over the top and not funny at all.

Despite the thunder in my ears and the fog that began blanketing my brain, I was able to grasp the story Neil relayed. He had been having strange symptoms: painful afternoon head-aches, a tunneling of his vision several times a day, and once or twice, a verbal response that was not normal—a slurring and jumble of words that didn't make sense. His girlfriend, Mia, a nurse, had become frightened, had said to him, "Did you hear what you said just now?" and insisted he go to her own doctor to be checked out. Her doctor had sent Neil for an MRI a day or two ago, had left him three messages today, and when Neil finally called back said, "Neil, your MRI has revealed that you have a serious brain tumor. You need to get someone to drive you to University-North Medical Center now."

"Tunneling" is a perfect description for what was happening to me as I pressed the phone against my ear. I took in fragments of phrases from a place beyond my usual sensory command station —"serious," "large," "eight centimeters," "in the car now with Mia," "I love you." And then his voice broke, and I could feel his tears more than hear them.

"Neil, I'll meet you there. Everything will be all right. I love you." And I hung up. I remember thinking how weird it was to just hang up—like a regular, routine call had just been completed. But there had been nothing left to do or say. It had all been said. Hanging on would have changed nothing, but hanging up sealed the deal. It had happened—the horrific phone call that is every parent's nightmare.

Like most parents, I had hoped, prayed to God, bargained with the Universe, figured that the odds were in my favor that a call like this one would never happen to me. But it had, on a cold night in January, when I was on retreat and completely alone.

And for what seemed like a very long time after letting go of my son's voice I sat with my eyes closed and my head hanging into my supporting hands, cradling myself. But the cradling supplied no comfort.

What finally roused me from the shock and inaction of my altered world were four little words charged with a message and a purpose, propelling me on then and in all the dark days to follow: "My baby needs me."

"My baby needs me" made it possible for me to contact Jim in Florida and experience the archetypal "WHAT?" from a new vantage point, for now I was the bearer of catastrophic news. It made it possible for me to phone Judy to drive me north through the dark winter night to University-North Medical Center to meet and hold my waiting son.

*n*AT THE TIME, MY SYMPTOMS didn't seem like a big deal to me. I had a slight case of tunnel vision every afternoon. At most, it would happen twice a day. The vision in my left eye would start to shrink and would continue until my sight in that eye would be closed off completely. In retrospect I see it as a big deal, but the whole thing would last a mere four seconds or so. Being twenty-eight and the worry-free kind of guy I was, I brushed it under the rug and told myself that I just needed a little more sleep and I would be fine. And I felt as fine as I always had.

Given this strange symptom, however, my girlfriend, Mia, a nurse, insisted that I see a doctor. Her concern began to scare me, and I decided the time had come to check things out. And this is where my story starts.

Dr. Rossi was a perfectly nice guy—late forties, fit, balding like me. I told him about the tunnel vision experiences. He seemed relatively unconcerned which picked up my spirits considerably. I knew we were blowing this whole thing out of proportion. Still, he thought it was a good idea to get an MRI to rule out the bad stuff. I had great health insurance through my teaching job so I thought, "Bring it on—let's get to the bottom of this." The appointment for the MRI was made before I left Dr. Rossi's office.

Ironically, I would joke about my tunnel vision happening because of a brain tumor. I remember talking myself into and out of the possibility of having a tumor, but I didn't really believe it. And joking about it classified it as lightweight and frivolous, but honestly, I think that deep down I was truly scared by such strange symptoms. Laughing about it took some of the fear out of the possibility.

In retrospect, I admit that I had more than just the tunnel vision symptom. I had had several severe headaches, and they had rattled me because of their intensity. The pain from these was very localized, always on the left side of my head.

In addition, twice during my afternoon math class another scary symptom appeared out of nowhere. I would be explaining the correspondence between decimals and percentages, and suddenly a really strange feeling would come over me. I had a sentence formed in my head, but when I tried to say it, nothing came out of my mouth. I couldn't articulate my thought. After a few seconds my ability to communicate would return, and I would finish the lesson. But that's when I decided I had to confide in Mia for her professional opinion.

Life at the Greenwood School where I was a teacher, soccer coach, and dorm head was always fast paced with forty-five learning disabled boys, many of them hyperactive as well. The day my MRI results were forwarded to Dr. Rossi's office was particularly busy for me. Besides my six A.M. wake-up duties and full schedule of classes, I was on afternoon duty—my turn to take charge of the students during faculty meeting. By the time I got back to my apartment in the late afternoon, I was exhausted. The MRI I'd had a few days before was the furthest thing from my mind.

I had left my cell phone at home that day. When I returned I flipped it open and noted a long list of missed calls from the same number, one I didn't recognize. I was about to call the mysterious number when the phone rang as I held it. It was Mia who sounded frantic.

"Neil," —she sounded breathy and rushed—"Dr. Rossi just called me. He said he's been trying to reach you all day. He wouldn't tell me what it was about, but I'm really scared it's something about your MRI."

"Mia, listen . . ." I did my best to sound calm. "Don't jump to scary conclusions. I just got in. I'll call him now and call you right back." We told each other "I love you."

I opened my phone again and noted that the missed calls were from a New Hampshire area code, the same area code as Dr. Rossi's office. All of a sudden I felt weak. Could my imaginary tumor be for real? My mind slid into dark places, but I reeled it back in. I told myself, "Just call the doctor and find out what's up."

I dialed the mysterious number though all the mystery had been rung out of it. When the receptionist put me through to Dr. Rossi, there was something in his voice that put me on guard. It's a bad feeling to have when you're calling for information on your MRI.

"Neil," he said slowly. "Normally I would never have this discussion outside of my office but, unfortunately, time is of the essence. Neil, the symptoms you've been experiencing are the result of a large tumor growing in your brain. You need to get up to University-North Medical Center immediately. They're expecting you."

I lost contact with his voice, his words. Although I remember hearing "eight centimeters," the conversation was over. And my worst scenario had happened. I had a confirmed brain tumor, and it was big.

When Mia arrived to pick me up, she was all efficiency and business, was assuming the familiar, professional role of a nurse who is trained to take charge, reminding me to grab my keys, my wallet, my cell phone, but I could see fear in her eyes.

Suddenly a clear thought pierced my confusion, my mental fog, and I was jerked into alertness. But the alertness was far worse than the fog because it added an extra layer of horror to the horror of the doctor's message. I had to tell my parents what was going on. And I would rather do anything else in the world—eat a can of worms, challenge a cheetah to a race, jump on a raging bull's back—than have to make that phone call telling my most loved ones that I had an eight centimeter tumor embedded in my brain.

Suddenly everything around me, myself included, was moving in slow motion. Moving on autopilot, I dialed my parents' number and heard my mom's familiar voice inviting me to leave a message—that she'd call back as soon as possible.

Knowing what I had to tell her made me nauseous. I waited for some words to come but when they didn't, I lost heart and hung up. I would do anything to protect my mom. And the only thing in my power at that moment was to put it off. I felt like a kid, hiding under the covers to save myself from the monster who was intent on finding me, cowering in my not-so-secret cave. But now, as always, the monster could never be tricked. I tried to swallow a growing lump in my throat and dialed the number again. I spit out a message, brief and urgent sounding. As I listened to myself I knew I sounded scared. And I knew my mom could always detect the slightest bit of worry or concern in my voice. But what could I do?

I rubbed the left side of my head and tried to shake off the shivers coursing through my body. The very idea of a tumor that could inevitably kill me growing inside my skull while I went about my daily life was creepy. But I had to stay focused. I hung up the phone, grabbed my stuff and followed Mia to the car.

As we headed north, I tried calling my parents again. Again, the answering machine was my only connection, and I reluctantly left another message. Where were my parents? It was getting late and they should be home by now.

Mia reached for my hand. "Neil," she said softly, "You're going to be all right." But something about the tight pressure of her hand did not reassure me.

Suddenly my phone rang and I jumped, my nerves in overdrive. The call was coming from my parents' phone. I answered and my mother's voice beamed across the miles that now separated us.

"Neil, it's me," I heard. "What's going on? What's wrong?"

I paused. "Mom, I want you to sit down for a minute." It was a corny line, I thought, even as I said it.

"Neil, what is it—you're scaring me!"

"Mom, I had an MRI two days ago. I have a brain tumor."

"What?!"—the sound of shock and disbelief.

"Mom, I'm on the way to University-North with Mia."

And finally, I broke down and started to cry. It just felt so good to hear my mother's voice. Suddenly I felt like a little boy again. All I wanted was to hold onto my mother. I needed to hide my face away from the world in her loving arms like I'd done when I was little.

"It's OK, Neil—you're going to be OK. I'm coming up right behind you, baby. Just hold on."

I hung up, my cheeks wet with the tears I'd held inside as long as I could. And Mia and I sped onward toward the hospital.

TWO

RECOLLECTIONS

"I feel a long way from where I began.
But I also feel a long way from where I am going."
~ Rachel Joyce

NEIL WAS BORN BLESSED IN MANY WAYS. It was his good fortune to be a twin whose womb mate was his companion through all the stages of early life and adolescence and who was his opposite and helpmate. Jackson was organized, linear, and responsible, as well as possessing a steady, sunny disposition. He kept our family on track by insuring that school permission slips were signed, library books returned on time, and information from his and Neil's day was relayed to us.

At eight weeks old, right on target, Jackson looked up at me and his sweet, round face broke into the widest, brightest smile. My heart melted with love and not a little pride. I loved milestones! And how could you not appreciate a baby who fulfilled the promise of the books on child development my friends and I were devouring in those days?

Neil arrived sunny, too, and with a special sparkle that attracted everyone. Charisma is not something you can specifically describe, but it almost oozes out of a person, and Neil had it, a magnetism that made others respond to him, a kind of social grace and inward knowledge of how to engage and charm people. But at eight weeks he was NOT gazing into my expectant face and charming me with his developmentally appropriately smile. In fact, he wasn't looking at me at all. He seemed to be gazing past me, somewhere "out there." I would stick my face close to his, many times a day, and he paid me no mind. I was sick.

About a week later, at a routine pediatrician appointment, with dread in my heart and my mind reeling with traumatic scenarios, I confessed my deep fear to our pediatrician: "I think this baby might be blind." The irony seems a little cruel to me today. Doctor Carmen was quiet. He did not quickly, categorically, allay my fear as I had hoped and expected. What I wanted to hear, I realized, was his reassurance that fraternal twins don't always develop in lock step. Instead, I thought I detected a shadow of worry cross his face. Mothers, after all, observe their babies like no one else. He turned off the light, reached for a flashlight, and swept it back and forth in front of Neil's eyes. And then he turned the light back on and faced me.

"Well, he doesn't track very well, but that flashlight sure excites him. He can see." I took Neil home, happy and relieved that my baby was normal. Silly me and my imagination.

Later that day, as I was standing across the kitchen from the twins' baby seats which I propped on the table as I prepared dinner, I noticed that Neil was looking toward me and following my movements. And it suddenly became clear to me that this small person focused outward. Jackson was examining the near details, and Neil was looking past us all to what was happening in the world beyond his reach.

And, indeed, Neil developed into a "global" type of guy. Attention to the details of life has never been his strength and has been a problem at times. He is spontaneous, generous, creative, warm, and fun—great qualities—but also the recipe for the kind of young man for whom growing up and becoming responsible can take awhile.

*n*AFTER GRADUATING FROM COLLEGE IN 2002, I wasn't ready to enter the real world, a place in my mind where you had to pay a hefty rent, start the long process of repaying student loans, show up from nine to five for a dreary job. No thanks. I wanted no part of it. I'd done what was expected of me, had accomplished what both my family and I had wanted: I'd graduated from college. Immediately afterward I headed for Utah to work as a lift operator at Alta, one of the foremost ski resorts in the United States. I envisioned a life traveling between the mountains and the sea, skiing and surfing my days away.

I'm sure my parents must have worried some about me and my long term plans, but at this point in my life I didn't think too far ahead. My immediate happiness was the goal. When I look back, I see myself as a race horse sporting blinders and only able to see what was immediately before me. I am oblivious to all the other horses to the right and left of me. I have no idea where I am racing to. I know that during this time I was not a very good person to the people I loved and who loved me—the fellowship of horses who ran by my side. Like many young people, I was floundering along. I had no inner knowledge of what I really wanted or was suited for. But a part of me knew, in a fuzzy kind of way, that there was more to life than the pleasure seeking I'd adopted as a life style.

When the ski season ended at Alta, I had to admit I could no longer live on the six dollars an hour I'd earned as a lift operator. I returned to Vermont with a half formed plan. I'd move into a rural compound with some of my boyhood friends and sock away some money by working at Prize Wholesale Groceries, a major employer in the area.

Prize is a huge warehouse which supplies food to major supermarkets in the northeast. The ground floor of the warehouse is about as large as six football fields with aisles and aisles of grocery items stacked at different levels under its sixty foot ceiling. I knew from growing up in the area that Prize is always hiring, that they paid $15.00 an hour for the first six months of working in the warehouse, and that those six months are considered the official training period. I could work a ten-hour a day shift and have a four-day work week. I submitted an application and was hired on as a grocery selector, a job many of us macho-type males would find downright entertaining, at least initially.

I got to drive a pallet-jack, a serious piece of industrial equipment that can go damn fast and be whipped around like a sports car despite its enormous weight. You drive in a standing position. Two forks protrude from the front of the jack and are long enough to hold two pallets, front to back. The name of the game for guys on the selector crew is to fill each pallet as fast as possible by referring, line by line, to the order sheet you have in hand. I'd check my sheet of stickers, drive to the designated aisle, jump off the jack, grab the item, slap the sticker on it, and eventually begin wrapping my collected items in cellophane to keep them from tumbling off the pallet as I'd race to the next location. Pallets were considered full when they reached about seven feet in height. Then I'd speed to the dock where my truck was being filled.

The reason for all this racing is due to the fact that the faster you go the more items you collect each hour. And that translates to the more money you make after your training period is over. This makes for a kind of cutthroat warehouse culture where you're top dog if you're the fastest. Everything depends on speed and competition. You always want to beat the next guy. Veteran selectors had no problem cutting you off and putting you in dangerous positions. You had to watch yourself when you dismounted your jack for an item. You ran the risk of accidentally being struck by a pallet jack flying by.

It didn't take long for me to feel wrung out by this job and the lifestyle I was living. For ten hours, four days a week, I didn't have time for an original thought or even a less than original one while I was on the clock. I was immersed in a frenzied existence, my focus being getting more and more proficient at quickly locating Gerbers Sweet Potato and Chicken # 45257867435.

What was I doing here? This was never in my life plan. I

never wanted to become a grocery selector. As a kid I'd wanted to become an air force test pilot; as an adolescent I'd longed to become a professional downhill mountain bike racer. Later, I'd toyed with the idea of becoming a teacher, probably a more realistic goal. During my college days I'd substitute taught in my mother's classroom when I was home from school, and it had struck a chord in me. I knew I was good in the classroom, but I hadn't gone down that road in college. So now I was stuck. Time was passing, and I was in a strange state of watching life go by. Why had I gotten a college degree? So I could efficiently lift boxes after applying the right sticker? I sure hoped not.

So, one morning, when I'd had enough, I quit my job at Prize, but I did it in the fashion that I did everything in those days: I just never showed up again. I collected my final check and never went back into the warehouse. I vowed to change my life, although a plan or a direction still eluded me. I just knew I'd be happier doing anything than working in a cave like Prize Wholesale Groceries.

As the seasons changed I longed to be outdoors. I felt that for a young guy like me it'd be crazy to work indoors during a Vermont summer when the whole world is vibrant with color and new life. I wanted to be front and center for the explosion of nature that happens here after months of neutral-colored lifeless-ness. So I took a job working for a close friend who is a brilliant stonemason and carpenter, and together we built some of the most beautiful stone walls in southern Vermont. We put in ten hour days of grueling but immensely satisfying work followed by cooking up huge portions of pasta for dinner and playing volleyball with friends until dark. I was busy and happy, with no time to ponder any long term goals.

Meanwhile, my mom had not given up on steering me in new directions. Our game had become predictable—she'd cast a lure and I would refuse to bite. But she never gave up on me, and, in the end, it was her persistence, her tenacity, that finally got me off my ass, out of my rut, and onto something new and empowering to my spirit.

One evening in late summer she called to let me know about a job opening she'd read about in the newspaper. She read me the brief job description over the phone: it was a part time position with strange hours—5:00 pm until 11:00 pm— at the Greenwood School, a boarding school for boys with learning problems, ages ten to sixteen, in neighboring Putney. She sounded excited and I, in turn, feigned excitement to please her. She asked if I might be interested in applying and if I wanted some help in sending in a resume and cover letter. We'd been down this road before, and because of my laziness and inability to follow through, I was sure this wasn't going to turn into anything, but I agreed.

We actually had fun as we worked together to create my first resume. It reminded me of the days when we'd worked on lesson plans the night before I'd substitute in her classroom. I sent the application in, and in short order I got a call from Greenwood to come in for an interview.

As I sat and chatted with the headmaster, I began to feel excited. I liked the way he described Greenwood as its own small community on the hill where all the faculty and staff worked together to make the school function smoothly. He told me they were looking for someone to arrive on campus at 5:00 to oversee evening activities. The boys would just be coming off of soccer practice and needed to shower, dress for dinner, and arrive on time. The prospective employee would have dinner with the students, return to the dorm to facilitate a block of free time, followed by study hall and preparation for bed. Bedtime duties included dispensing medications to students who were diagnosed with attention deficit disorder, hyperactivity, or Asperger's Syndrome, a mild form of autism. After reading a quick story to the younger boys it would be "lights out" time. When everyone was settled in, the employee would remain in the Common Room, relaxing or reading until the two dorm heads would assume responsibility at 11:00.

The day after my interview I was offered the job, and I accepted immediately. And that decision had a huge impact on my life.

Initially, I worked my carpentry-masonry job for the first stretch of every day, leaving a little early to make it to the Greenwood campus by 5:00. It amazed me that I looked forward to starting that second job each day. It made me feel so good to show up at the dorm and have the boys be delirious with excitement just to see me and know that I was in charge for the next five hours. The job gave me energy I didn't know I had. It made me feel alive again, a memory that brings me to tears when I think back on it all. I was finally in a place where I felt at home, where I believed my life was, at last, going in a direction that had been waiting for me.

I found myself in a space that allowed me to reflect on myself through the work I was doing. I learned that for learning disabled students a predictable daily schedule makes a huge difference in their ability to function and succeed. And I saw that this was equally true for me. The structure of our days kept me calmer and more efficient. I had a lot more in common with these boys than I'd ever recognized.

I used to think that being in the right place at the right time was a chapter in the book of Old Wives Tales, meaning it wasn't really true, but I've changed my mind because it happened to me. Not that long after I started my part-time job at Greenwood, a teacher, who also happened to be one of the two dorm heads, left in the middle of the year. He and the job didn't fit well, and Greenwood was temporarily stuck. And there I was, waiting in the wings, ready to go when I was offered the job. I couldn't believe my good luck! Practically overnight I was a full-time employee with a heavy load. I became a dorm head, soccer coach, and math teacher at a school I already knew and loved. I totally appreciated their vote of confidence and was confident, deep within me, that I wouldn't let them down. I'd already bonded with the boys and had made strong connections with some of the neediest. Now, as first floor dorm head, I felt like a surrogate father. I loved those kids like they were my own.

I moved into the apartment off the Common Room to be available and in charge, not only during daytime hours but all night as well. And more than a few times a scene like this would occur: I would be sleeping peacefully when my doorbell would ring. I'd drag myself out of bed and open the door to a little guy, his face red and swollen from crying. He'd look up at me and say, "Neil—I'm homesick." It would break my heart. Suddenly I'd be transported back to my own childhood, and I could feel the homesickness I'd felt, awake in my cabin at camp, alone in the dark.

"I know how that feels, buddy," I'd say, and with my heart properly melted I'd find the energy to make hot chocolate at 3:30 in the morning. We'd sit in the Common Room and talk about our families and how he would be seeing his in a very short time.

~

It was so ironic that I ended up becoming a math teacher. And because of that twist of fate I grew in ways I never could have imagined. I could relate to my students' hatred of all things involving math because I'd been the same way. I had a history of going blank as soon as math class began. I had no interest in it and showed no particular skill with it. But because of my own experience, my own struggles, I became a very good math teacher to those boys. I wanted things to be different for them. I worked hard at coming up with a variety of ways to look at a problem. My methods included hands-on activities to supplement or take the place of the purely symbolic presentation of problem solving, and I set problems into a story model. I invented recurring characters, like Gramma Tillie who was always getting herself into trouble and could only be rescued by using a math function we were working on.

"Come on boys," I'd say, "this is your grandma. Be her hero!"

I play-acted and they interacted and math became more understandable, more fun, than either they or I could have anticipated.

~

I would have to say now, in retrospect, that although I was coming into my own with the beginning of a life plan that excited and nurtured me, there were times I felt "off" and wondered what was wrong with me. I was handling my responsibilities at Greenwood, was a favorite of the students, received compliments from the parents, so why was I often anxious? My mother felt that I had become "distant" during our times together as a family. And many times I had let them down by not showing up when I said I would, by not following through on projects I'd promised to get done. I could not deny my behavior, but I couldn't put my finger on the source of the problem. At times I would feel a moment of clarity—feel that the answer was ready to present itself—but it didn't. And the moment would pass, and the sensation of knowing would fade away. I would return to my life, feeling like I was missing something but not knowing what it was.

*a*THERE HAS ALWAYS BEEN A CLOSENESS between Neil and me and here's why: we are twins of a sort—not the actual, physical twin-ness that he shares with his brother, of course—but we are twins by nature, by style, by strengths and weaknesses. He inherited much of me, the good and the bad.

That makes the bond between us tight; it also makes the frustrations I feel for our shared flaws very intense.

Because of this natural connection, I had to take very seriously my intuition that something was not right with Neil at some point in his twenties. He had been a happy, free-wheeling child, a warm and dynamic youth. He had finished college on schedule, but over time, there were parts of him that felt foreign to me. And it was not just over-anxious me who recognized that the spacey, somewhat disorganized qualities of Neil had intensified into not being able to finish a project, tuning out, and more than the usual impatience. His older sister shared my concern, confirmed all that I felt, and validated that I was not crazy, over critical, or simply disappointed in the direction in which Neil was headed as a person and family member.

But what could we do? Over a couple of years time, several letters went back and forth between Neil and me about keeping his word and being the man of honor that his father had modeled for him all his life. He would respond to me with agreement, obvious reflection, and promises of not letting me down—of being the man that I knew he could be. It was not an easy time for us, and like many, maybe the majority of moms and twenty-something-year-olds, we kept our distance and talked less frequently. "Nothing wrong with that," I told myself. "What young person doesn't need privacy and space to develop and explore?"

And there were, without a doubt, good signs and positive developments. Most heartening was his entering the teaching field and his excitement over his experiences and successes in that world. But I found myself wondering, in retrospect, whether Neil's seeming personality change was due to the tumor which grew to the size of a small orange, pushed his brain to one side of his skull, and, for a time, robbed him of the "Neilness" I knew and loved.

THREE

WAITING GAME

Sitting here in limbo
Waiting for the dice to roll
Sitting here in limbo
Got some time to search my soul.

~ Jimmy Cliff

*n*AN HOUR AND A HALF AFTER we set off from Brattle-boro, Mia and I arrived at University-North Medical Center. We hurried out of the early evening cold and into the warmth of the hospital. We made our way to the Emergency Room and found it packed with people. "This might take awhile," I thought to myself.

Mia grabbed my hand and led me to the front desk. The receptionist asked my name and date of birth, and Mia began providing the information while I stood right next to her. Even in my spacey state, it rubbed me the wrong way—as if my tumor had suddenly changed me, and I could no longer answer simple questions. I interrupted Mia and took charge myself.

The receptionist clicked into her computer, looked back up at me and said, "Neil, we are expecting you. Stay right here—we'll have a nurse show you to an exam room."

I was caught off guard when a nurse quickly emerged from

the back and led Mia and me to a small, curtained cubicle. Why was I going to the front of such a long line of other people waiting to be seen? Suddenly I felt sick to my stomach again. The gravity of the situation was becoming clearer to me.

The nurse handed me a pair of drawstring pants and a pajama top with tie strings at the back. Mia helped me into the top and tied it for me. Little did I know this would be my outfit for the next two months—the dreaded patient's outfit.

I sat, waiting, on the edge of the exam table. Mia leaned against the wall, my MRI disk which we had picked up before driving north in her hand. It looked so plain and innocent as she held it. Looking at her, I imagined she was about to pop that CD into the player in my apartment to introduce me to her new favorite song. Wouldn't that be so much more believable than all this insanity? There had to be some kind of mistake. They must have mixed up someone else's results with mine. That was it. Or just maybe I'd shut my eyes for a moment and was in the middle of a dreadful nightmare.

The curtain swished open, breaking the silence. And, once again, I had to confront the reality of my situation. Two doctors—or what I assumed were doctors as they were both wearing white coats and stethoscopes—walked in. We all exchanged handshakes before they took seats and invited Mia to join us in a half circle. The younger of the two asked me how I was feeling, whether I was currently on any medication, if I had suffered any seizures. God, no, of course not! He took my blood pressure and pulse and the older man asked if they could have the MRI we'd brought with us. Mia handed it to him and he loaded it into the computer. I watched as an image of my brain appeared on the screen.

At first everything looked fine to me, but I had no idea how magnetic resonance imagining works. I was looking at the first picture, taken from the top of my brain, without realizing that there were many images to follow due to the machine's ability to scan down the skull and reveal deeper recesses. Imagine my head as a pumpkin being sliced a hundred times by a sharp knife or samurai sword, thinly and horizontally. Each slice is exactly parallel to the last. Only the device doing the sectioning is a camera.

As the doctors began to scan lower, toward the middle of my brain, things started to look bad—really bad. All of the symptoms I had experienced and foolishly ignored—the localized headaches, the tunnel vision, the short befuddled gaps of speech I'd experienced in my classroom—well, now I was staring at the reason for them on a computer screen in a major teaching hospital on a frigid winter evening. And it was not a pretty picture.

The doctor paused on the image of the tumor at its largest. It was imposing, to say the least. It was obviously a growth that was very different from the normal brain material. It didn't take a trained eye to see this. It looked like a knot or a burl growing in a tree, an anomaly that is out of sync with the proper way that wood should grow. This tumor had grown to such a size that it was squeezing my brain out of its rightful place. It laid claim to the left hemisphere of my cranium, pushing all the good stuff into the right, making for a very tight fit.

The younger of the men got overly excited at this point, almost to the point of being unprofessional. His questions became fervent. How could my symptoms have been as intermittent as

I'd reported? How was my balance? My vision? The symptoms I'd described didn't seem to reflect a tumor of this significance. It was like the guy had never seen a growth like this before. Then the two of them left the room. I guessed that they were conferring.

Have you ever been in a situation when, suddenly, it feels as though all the oxygen has been sucked out of the room? You feel short of breath, as if you had just sprinted beyond your capacity and it's possible you could faint? For me, sitting helpless in that curtained cubicle, everything seemed to dim in the looming reality of what we had just seen. Mia and I were left alone in a darker space than we had entered.

How could I hold onto any hope after seeing that MRI? Before I could even work with the question, however, the older doctor came back into the room. Mia had to jostle my arm because I didn't realize that he was asking me a question. I was staring off into space. All I heard was that the tumor was about the size of an orange. I remember trying to get my mind around that fact. How could my brain continue to live around this massive growth? I felt numb and wished I could feel even more numb.

"Can you contact your family," the white coat asked me, "to let them know you're being admitted to the hospital tonight?" Mia began to answer for me again. The doctor didn't seem to mind. And, I thought to myself, "To hell with it—neither do I."

*a*I'VE ALWAYS BEEN OVERLY SQUEAMISH. There was never a blood and guts trauma in my earlier life that would account for my aversion to most medical issues, but I definitely have a major sensitivity. Strangely, I'm not squeamish regarding worms in the garden, or snakes, if I see them before being startled by their presence. I was even incredibly brave during the summers while my kids and their friends were growing up and spending happy days playing in our stream which got typically lazy in August. They'd arrive at the back door, saying, "Mom, I need the salt—leeches are stuck to me." I would nonchalantly hand them the box so they could petrify those creepy, black parasites. However, a squished mouse in a trap sends me squealing. I just hate "gory."

But what mother doesn't witness her share of childhood accidents in the raising of three children? Of course I didn't escape those experiences, but luckily I always got to play the supporting role in jumping to action. Jim, who had taken some EMT courses, was a natural at ministering to on-site emergencies. My role was to avert my eyes, call ahead to the emergency room, and be the driver. I always felt that I was an important contributor, and I never had to admit how relieved I was that I never had to actually, you know— "look."

So it was not in the least surprising that I simply refused to look at the computer screen in the emergency room of University-North Medical Center upon my arrival that January night in order to verify the large mass in the left hemisphere of Neil's brain. Everyone else seemed morbidly interested: the intern, my helpmate Judy who was posing as my stepsister in order to gain admittance with me, Neil's girlfriend Mia, even Neil himself. If, indeed, seeing is believing, then I could understand how that

MRI image was an important focal point in that tiny cubical—backing up those unbelievable, unbearable words with graphic, visual proof.

I cannot recall the words spoken by those interns from Neurology that evening, but I got the message: it was bad. And it was big. Neil told me later that they expressed their amazement that he was walking, talking, and functioning at all.

I looked at my six foot two inch son, stretched out on the emergency room bed with his head propped up on a pillow, and he seemed just fine to me—just like regular Neil—and he gazed around at all of us with a kind of shy and apologetic smile and said, "I just don't know what to say." And this part IS indelibly etched into my memory. I walked over to him, wrapped my arms around him and said, "Neil—you are surrounded by love." And he whispered back to me, "I can feel it."

How was it possible that Neil had taught school just this morning and now, at day's end, was being admitted to the Neurology unit to await whatever the next step would be? My mind began to turn in on itself. I felt as though I was standing by my own side, not fully connected to the "me" whose skin I'd been comfortable in just hours earlier. Tomorrow, I knew, would be completely unfamiliar, surreal. It wasn't possible to even imagine what it would be like. Our family, not even fully assembled yet, would be facing an emergency—that much I "got." But beyond that, everything was a black screen.

It was a given that Mia would spend the night with Neil. I would return home to figure out what to do regarding my teaching job and get ready to be fully present for Neil the next day. I told him I would be back early in the morning after I made arrangements at home, and I remember walking down a long dark corridor with Judy as she spoke to her husband on the phone. "Yes—he has a very large brain tumor. I saw the MRI. He's been admitted and we are on our way back."

One more nail in the coffin of "New Reality," and I couldn't comprehend whose life they were talking about. It just couldn't be mine. It couldn't be Neil's. It couldn't be our family's. Most of the way back through that black winter night we didn't speak. I heard a sort of mewing inside the car, like a cat in pain—maybe trapped in a hole or nursing a shattered limb—and I knew it was coming from me, a primal, guttural response to a mind gone numb.

As we pulled into my driveway, Judy asked if I wanted her to stay. And I said no, I'd be OK, there were things I needed to do. Deep down I knew there was nothing in the world anybody could do to help me. I was lost, had disappeared to a place where even a hand extended to me in compassion could not help —might even make me scream—because it was incapable of saving me, of hauling me up over the cliff. "The Call," the nightmare, had happened, and all the rehearsing and morbid "what if" anticipating that was hard-wired inside me had not made me more fit and able to deal.

So what did I do, all alone on that cruel night of January 31, 2008? I cleaned. I reorganized the mudroom entryway of our house, separating winter shoes and boots to be put on the shoe shelf from non-winter ones destined for the closet. The task became very important as I methodically set to work. The day before, I had tossed the footwear into a hodge-podge pile waiting to be sorted. Now, even in my altered state, I recognized that if anyone saw this mess in my absence, I would be embarrassed. Tying up loose ends that night was a form of caring for myself. I had no control over what had just happened and no inkling of what the days ahead would look like. But I did have the power to clean up a mess of shoes. Engaging in something mundane, homely, and familiar was a salve for my mind battered by shock. I could rest it for a spell, float on automatic pilot, and allow some clear thinking to rise to the surface.

And so it was that I made a plan to stop by my school early the next morning, well before opening, to relay my family's emergency to the secretary and principal and give them adequate time to arrange for a sub. I also recognized that I must lie down and take some rest before facing whatever lay ahead.

AS SOON AS I WAS ADMITTED and settled into a room on the Neurology floor, I phoned Jackson to fill him in on the surreal turn my life had taken. After we hung up he drove through the night from New York City to be by my side. My sister Jessica from North Carolina arrived early that evening. She and my father, who had caught the earliest flight he could from Florida, had connected at the airport in Connecticut and drove to New Hampshire together in a blinding snow. It seemed so ironic to me that as we all sat together on my hospital bed I felt strong and healthy. It felt as though I was playing hookey or that somehow I'd created a big hoax. I had gathered my family together—everyone was here because of me—and I was fine. But I knew I wasn't. And having them and Mia here in this strange room, a room I was told I needed to be in, did make me feel that I was surrounded by love.

My memories of the days that followed are like a patchwork quilt not completely stitched together. Each piece is an individual moment or day, and some of them are more vivid than others. Sometimes, even now, I will rediscover several of the pieces and reattach them to the quilt that is my memory. Other times, patches that I thought were securely attached have come loose and fallen away.

It didn't take long to learn from the neurosurgeons that surgery was the necessary next step. At this point, my family went into a hyperactive state of research. While University-North has an outstanding reputation, none of us knew if it was the best place to deal with my particular predicament. As testament to the cohesiveness of my family, everyone became involved in one way or another. My father, an inveterate on-line investigator, holed up in the hospital library to research brain tumors and the most current methods of treatment. My mother, sister, and girlfriend looked into hospitals that were recommended to them by those who had some knowledge of brain tumors or some story of others who had needed to find this information for themselves or loved ones.

While all this happened around me, I went about my days falling in and out of sleep, playing YouTube music with Jackson, and taking phone calls from friends. I was living in a haze. While all the decisions that were being considered were relevant and even interesting to me, I would think about them for a few minutes and then become disconnected. I couldn't stay focused. I felt on the periphery of it all. I heard and took part in conversations but had a hard time grasping it was me this was all about. A couple of days ago everything was rosy. Now I didn't know up from down.

Ultimately, my family decided it was best to stay where we were for the surgery, and I agreed. I had no desire to pick up and move from a hospital others traveled far and wide to come to. So the plan was set, but the waiting continued. The neurosurgeon who was the most experienced and most skilled at performing the particular type of surgery I needed was away at a conference when I was admitted. When he returned, it took a couple of days to assemble a team and schedule an operating room. I remember wishing I could just be operated on immediately—this very day—as my mind couldn't help but plunge me into very dark places. What if I just never woke up? What if I woke up with full control of my mind and my entire body was paralyzed? Or the reverse—my body survived and my mind was gone?

I did my best to appear upbeat, and, of course, I was grateful beyond measure for all the love and support surrounding me. Trying my hardest to lighten the load of those who loved me—that, I recognized fairly quickly—was the task I needed to take on.

EARLY THAT MORNING, AS I pulled into the parking lot of University-North Medical Center, I saw my New York son,

Jackson, standing with Mia. He had driven through the night, arrived at some ungodly hour, and now the two of them were stretching their limbs and taking in some fresh air after spending long hours in Neil's room. Mia had slept as best she could in the reclining chair next to Neil's hospital bed.

Seeing one of my children or Jim, especially when I am taken by surprise by their unexpected presence, has always been like a miracle drug to me. Something about that wide Taylor smile or a particular quality of energy they emanate turns on a light inside me, and I fell into Jackson's arms with gratitude. He was here for his twin brother, but I, too, needed him beside me.

Neil was settled into a large, private, light-filled room in Neurology with a beautiful view of the New Hampshire woodland. He had already enchanted the nurses with his warmth and winning sense of humor They had discovered that despite his size and athletic build he is what is commonly called a "hard stick." His veins are thin and deeply embedded and almost impossible to implant an I.V. line into on the first or second try. At one point, as a nurse approached him with the usual paraphernalia, Neil responded, "I think you and I both know this isn't going to work, but, hey, give it your best shot." She laughed.

It started to snow. As the snow collected outside the window, I worried about the trip that Jim and Jessica were making from Florida and North Carolina. I figured they would make it into Bradley International in Connecticut, but the long drive north to New Hampshire would most likely be slow and treacherous.

I don't remember a day in which the hours crawled along so slowly as that February 1st. There was nothing to do but worry about everything. We were in grave trouble, and we didn't know what the next step was—had no one, so far, to guide us, no choices to make, no journey to even contemplate beginning. If there is a hell, or that holding place called Hades, this had to be a dead ringer for it.

The neurosurgeon who had been the first to speak to us about Neil's tumor pretty much admitted that he was not the doctor to perform this particular brain surgery, and although I didn't feel a connection with him, it increased my panic. His message seemed to be, "This is no piece of cake operation." He was going to refer the case to the chief of Neurology, but he was away at a conference and had several surgeries scheduled upon his return.

There were times that day when Neil asked Jackson to call his friends, especially his two closest friends in Colorado and California. These requests made the situation brutally real to Neil, and he would start to cry. I'd wrap my arms tightly around him, but my feelings of helplessness were like none I'd ever experienced. At other times, Neil and Jackson would be on the computer for long periods, surfing YouTube for their favorite music and taking turns making selections. They appeared to be totally normal and natural—as if we were simply on a weekend outing together. From time to time we would leave the room to visit the upscale cafeteria, view the art exhibits in the hallways, listen to a musician play the grand piano in the downstairs lobby, and just learn the lay of the land. As the never ending day wore on, my ability to function and to stay present began to deteriorate, and I felt a powerful need to withdraw into a cave-like space. Late that afternoon I gave into this need in a way that I continued all my days at University-North Hospital. I made a pallet using a folded blanket and a pillow on the hard floor of the hospital room. I lay down and covered myself, including my head, with a second blanket, and mummy-like, fell into a state that looked like simple sleep but was different in some way. It was a deeper loss of consciousness, a brief drug-like state that provided some respite from despair and, upon awakening, made it possible for me to get up and keep going.

And so it was that I was cocooned in my very first pallet when the door opened and Jim and Jessica walked in, bringing their light, their love, their support, and their added resources. The beam of their combined energy went right to Neil, and how could I not feel that everything in this moment was so much better than it had been a few moments earlier, and how even in a time like this, some respite is possible.

~

As Day Number One of our surreal new reality was winding down, Jackson and I were sent out to find a place for us to stay. We had a list of motels that offered special reduced prices to the families of patients who were being treated at University-North. Jim had instructed us to make reservations for the next three nights. As we headed out it struck me how obvious this mission was—and how it had not entered my own mind. I wondered when it would have dawned on me to take action and face the facts? Our entire life had left home and shifted to out of town, where we would remain not for three nights but for what seemed like endless weeks.

Despite the anguish of those days, when I think back to our time at the Days Inn, it is with warmth and gratitude for the friendly and respectful shelter it offered us when we so needed some comfort, the diversion of TV, and a therapeutic beer in order to recharge for whatever awaited us the following day.

~

With the troops rallied, it was decision time. We needed a solid game plan with delineated steps to follow in order to ground us, to keep us from floating out into directions that beckoned and pulled us but were confusing and unclear. It was on our radar that the premier medical center for dealing with brain cancer was The University of North Carolina Medical Center where Ted Kennedy had just undergone surgery and treatment for his brain cancer, an event that, due to his fame and prestige, received much publicity. We knew that time was an important factor for Neil, and plans were not coming together in a timely manner at University-North. We were desperate to move forward, to feel more proactive and less helpless.

Jim retreated to the hospital library to research young men and brain tumors, a grim task, the facts of which he would not share with me. Jackson's job was to be there one hundred percent for Neil—to keep him from slipping down the slope of panic and despair. Mia, Jessica, and I called North Carolina and conferred with the University-North social worker who coordinated the sending off of Neil's MRI and other essential reports to the doctors down south. We worked at a desperate, feverish pace, not having a clue if the idea of transferring hospitals really made sense, was workable for us as a family, or was the medically right decision. I think it dawned on me, somewhere down this road, that if leaving New Hampshire was the choice we made, then not all of us would be present for Neil's surgery. Jackson and Mia, most certainly, would not be able to completely suspend their work lives to follow Neil south. And they were essential members of the team. Despite my confusion about our next step, I plugged away at the necessary details of preparing for a possible transfer. It felt important to explore all options.

During this time, we would take Neil out of the hospital with us. Living in limbo is boring as well as stressful. We needed relief from the hospital environment, and he still seemed fine. Going out to dinner offered a break from our woes. For a while we could pretend that we were a normal family choosing where we wanted to sit at Margarita's Restaurant along with all the other patrons living normal lives. I remember wondering one evening about other dinner outings in my life, when I was whole and unburdened and free from pain. Who around me then had been harboring a sad secret, a terrifying diagnosis, unbeknownst to fellow diners just a table away? Now it was our turn—we were those other people, and I knew exactly how it felt.

~

Late one afternoon, a man I'd never seen before, in hospital scrubs, appeared at our door—and I say "our" door, as Neil's room was now the Taylor family encampment—and introduced himself as Dr. Carrington, the chief of neurology.

For some reason, I was completely taken by surprise. It was almost as if I didn't quite believe that Dr. Carrington existed. But here he was now in the flesh—trim, bespectacled, gray haired, and soft-spoken with the kind of easy manner that confident people seem to unconsciously display. We fell in love with him on the spot. Dr. Carrington was ready to schedule Neil's surgery. He was also perfectly willing to help us make arrangements at another hospital of our choosing. He knew the North Carolina surgeons, as brain surgery, he told us, is not a highly populated profession; most doctors in the field know each other. He seemed confident in his own abilities and his place in the field. He was not looking for business. He had a busy case load, as people from out of the area often sought out University-North for treatment.

Dr. Carrington wanted us to understand that Neil's brain tumor, as revealed on the MRI, was serious business. He outlined the procedure he would undertake if he was to become Neil's surgeon. He would use the brain mapping technique Jim had recently read was the best and most current method of brain surgery. During the operation Neil would be awake, as there are no pain centers within the brain. The team would speak to Neil in order to pinpoint the safest way to cut and remove the tumor without doing damage to the functional centers of the brain. He felt that he would be able to safely remove about ninety percent of the tumor; the rest would be dealt with using radiation and, if it proved to be malignant, chemotherapy.

I think that during Dr. Carrington's explanation Jim and I may have exchanged glances, but I knew intuitively what Jim was thinking—here is our doctor, here is our hope, here is our plan, and here is some relief from the constant mind-spin of "what do we do?" Without excusing ourselves for a family consultation, Jim asked Dr. Carrington to sign on and to schedule Neil's surgery as soon as possible. We would stay here at University-North, close to our home and everything we knew.

To me, "as soon as possible" meant NOW, in an hour, the next morning after the doc got a good eight hours and a strong cup of joe. But I guess hospitals don't exactly work that way. It's important to know that you actually have an operating room available and a team who knows they are expected, with some prior notice. So Dr. Carrington indicated that the surgery would take place in two to three days time.

After he left, we high-fived—Neil, Jim, Jackson, Jessica, Mia, and me. Happiness is the strangest phenomenon—it's a total surprise to witness its rise during grim times when the heart feels crushed under a rock, and you just know it will be pinned there permanently. The rock will never give way and roll off. But here we were, graced with some movement, and good cheer rose in all of us. To celebrate, we decided to head into town to have dinner at a fun and funky little restaurant on Main Street, very close to the university. One of Jackson's college buddies who was finishing a graduate program at the university would join us. Life was looking better. And we were still our own agents.

We had been told by the nursing staff that while no one could stop us, it was not recommended that Neil leave the hospital. Despite having been put on anti-seizure medication the moment he'd been admitted, he was still at risk for seizure due to the size and location of his tumor. While this was a sober warning, we chose not to heed it. We put our faith in the meds and focused instead on Neil's emotional well being. Wasn't it our job to keep him focused on the positive? How better to do this than by taking him out in the world to do everyday happy things? This was the primary mission of our team, to let him know that we believed he would come through this, that we would all live through it together, and that brighter days lay ahead. This would end up being a distant nightmare, a test that we would pass and be the stronger for it.

The restaurant was a dimly lit, cozy retreat from the relentless cold. It was buzzing with parka-clad, athletic looking young people and fit, well-heeled older patrons. Rather than table cloths, each table was covered with a sheet of brown paper and held a jar of crayons and markers for diners to doodle with while waiting for their food to arrive. And so we set to work, with laughter and high spirits. More that one of us drew funny, endearing little caricatures of Dr. Carrington, our newest team member, the person who had just brightened our day. But as hard as we tried, there was still, for me, that lump in my throat—always there. I couldn't detect that bleak place in the others as we sat together, but I could see that Neil was somewhat quiet and withdrawn. He wasn't completely on board. There was part of him that seemed distant, shut down, somewhere else.

I realized that night that we, his team, could stand on the banks of the flood waters that had become our joint life, reach our arms out to grab and hold him, but in the end, this was his journey. We were the ones who remained high and dry. I know for myself, as his mother, who loved him more than life, that if I could have dived in and swapped places, I would have done so in a heartbeat. But that was not a choice available to me.

~

The Waiting Game continued for a couple more days. It included many supportive phone calls from friends and family and Neil's work colleagues, dozens and dozens of cards, the most endearing from Neil's young students, and gifts of money to help us during this time of living away from home. The private school where Neil worked expressed its love for him, emotionally and financially. We were humbled by their caring and generosity. The outpouring of support also, at times, felt like a cattle prod confirming that this crisis was actually happening. I knew it was, because others were verifying it with fruit baskets and flowers and messages of support and concern. It was not just pretend, a nasty dream, a TV drama. This was real and we had to deal with it.

Two brief conversations I had with Neil during those long, blurry days will be with me always, for they foreshadowed the brave and wise being who was forced to be born anew in the winter of 2008. One took place in his hospital room. I remember him stretched out on the bed and me standing over him, our hands entwined. He said, "One thing I can't deal with is a scary thought that keeps whirling around in my mind. What if I can never ride my mountain bike again?"

I looked at this extreme-athlete son of mine and calmly said, "Neil, I'm sure you will ride your mountain bike again. But if for some reason you can't, you'll find something else—you'll swim, or whatever."

And he said, "Yeah, you're right."

In the other vignette we are walking together from the hospital food court back to his room, a daily ritual we took in various groups. Neil and I are alone, and he looks down at me and said, "Mom, whatever happens will be all right."

Some quiet energy in him, physically, passed into me in an instant. My breathing seemed to change from jagged and a-rhythmic to calm and even.

"Do you really feel that Neil?"

He answered without pause, "Yes, I do. "

As we wound our way down the now familiar hallway, I held his hand against my cheek—oh, my precious boy. I told him again, like I did every day, "You are surrounded by love."

∽

Being in a state of suspension when all you want to do is move forward, act, and "fix" things is very trying. Time becomes thick and heavy and hard to deal with. You feel submerged, with no skill or strategy to overcome the unrelenting sluggishness of slow motion. That's when rescue is so important. That is when angels, in the guise of ordinary people, can transform your experience just by being who they are and offering what they have to give. Their path crosses yours, and the intersection sparks light and energy into your life. Neil had two such experiences during his days before surgery, both prompted by private visits.

The first was a visit from Karen Robinson, the hospital social worker. She was immensely helpful to our family in many ways, both emotionally and practically. Other, religiously affiliated personnel from the hospital had approached us, having recognized or been told that we were in trouble, but Jim would have none of them. Karen Robinson was different. She was compassionate in a humanistic way, knowledgeable about services available, and had helped us through the drudgery of paperwork. She was wise, straight-forward, and knew the ins and outs of family life in a hospital setting.

She made an appointment with Neil one afternoon, and they met alone in his room. They spent a long time together. Neil, to my knowledge, had never before met with a therapist, but I guess it was not hard for him to express his feelings, his fears. He seemed peaceful when I entered his room after her departure. He told me that their time together had been very meaningful to him—had made him feel calmer and more centered. Not only did he like Karen, but he had had a chance to glimpse her world, her profession, her skill in situations such as his. He was impressed with what she brought to him, taught him.

Karen didn't share any specifics of the experience with me except to tell me what an amazing person Neil was. And I remember thinking, "Thank God—only an amazing person could stay the steady course." And Neil seemed to be doing that. Amazing.

The second visit came by way of a gift from Neil's aunts, Jane and Jean. They decided to send a massage therapist to his hospital room, hoping that body work before his surgery would relax his mind as well as soothe and prepare his body. I was grateful that Neil would have another diversion, something to help eat up the hours before his date in the operating room. To me, that was an equally important aspect of their gift.

At the prescribed hour, there was a knock on the door and in walked a youngish man, one I never would have taken for a massage therapist. I guess I must have harbored a stereo-type—physically fit, tall, cool. The gift sent to Neil was short, overweight, and wearing Bermuda shorts on a February afternoon in New Hampshire. Go figure. Despite my less than confident first impression, he seemed amiable, chatty, sure of himself, and I was impressed that he immediately focused on Neil and Neil's situation. I beat a hasty retreat thinking, "Neil is not going to relate to this guy. But, hey, this is not my gift. I can't control everything, and the silver lining is that I get an hour to myself." As I walked down that now-too-familiar hallway, however, it dawned on me that being alone with me was a debatable gift this winter of 2008.

When I re-entered Neil's room after an hour had passed, I found him blissful. Naturally, I was curious. How had this quirky massage guy worked a measure of magic? I will never know, but Neil said it was an amazing hour of bodywork and deep connection on many levels. None of the particulars mattered to me, but it seemed like a gift from the Universe, channeled by the aunties. There was no way I could have foreseen that that hour was a turning point in Neil's life and a living testament to the age old saying, "When one door closes, another opens."

*n*I'D NEVER HAD A MASSAGE before, but when my aunts phoned to say they'd arranged for a massage therapist to come to my hospital room, I was excited. And, OK, I'll admit I envisioned a buff, female working her magic on my now over-stressed body.

When I answered the knock at the appointed time, however, I was face to face with a short, chubby man who asked if I was the one awaiting a massage. My house of cards collapsed on the spot as I realized that this was the massage therapist and not her driver, as I had hoped. "Yes sir, I'm the one," I answered. He nodded and entered the room.

Around his waist was a fanny pack which I soon learned held his massage oil, and he was lugging a large but lightweight, portable table. "He must be aiming for a workout," I thought, because he was wearing a pair of gym type shorts despite the frigid temps. Who would wear shorts in February in New Hampshire? In about three seconds he had unclipped the table, unfolded it, popped the legs out, and deftly flipped it into position. As I watched him stretch a sheet over the table, something he'd probably done a million times, I noted that he moved around the table efficiently, even gracefully. He turned to me and introduced himself, and I did the same.

"Well, Neil, it is a pleasure to meet you. Why don't you get undressed as I finish up here." I slid out of my hospital garb and stood in my underwear as he finished putting the top sheet on the table. And then he focused all his attention on me.

"All right, Neil. We're all set. Get under the top sheet and lie face down with your face supported by the headrest."

He spoke in a soft but confident voice, and never having had a massage before I really appreciated the instructions. He asked if I was comfortable with the setting of the headrest, and, surprisingly, I felt more comfortable than I had in a long time.

I can't tell you exactly what happened during the next hour, but the massage I got from John—the whole experience he provided—transcended anything I ever imagined about massage. I certainly regretted the superficial thoughts I'd had about what kind of shape I thought John was in. What a jerk I can be!

It was almost like time slowed down. I AAAhhhed and OOOooooed throughout the session, and I found that I wanted to or needed to talk. And John was completely open to that. In fact, he was a gifted conversationalist, so intelligent and sincere that I felt great trust in him. I told him my whole story and admitted how very scared I was. He listened quietly, then asked me all the right questions. I felt as though I was with an old friend I could tell anything to. In the course of an hour, he skillfully found all the knots, all the hot spots, all the trigger points in my body. Even as we talked, his fingers manipulated my muscles and connective tissue the way a master violinist's fingers must dance across the strings.

It was a miracle and a blessing that for an hour under John's healing touch I was released from the dark thoughts of the possibility of dying. I slowly got up off the table feeling like a new man. I gave John a huge hug and told him how much the last hour meant to me, how gifted he was, how heavenly the whole experience had been. He hugged me back and wished me the best.

As I watched him pack up, it felt strangely as if my best friend was leaving, even though I had known him for all of one hour. I remember telling myself, "After everything that lies ahead, you might lose a million beautiful memories, but hold onto this one." And I have. I felt as though I had emerged from the fog I had been living in since my diagnosis. I felt strong and ready to take on the world, even though that meant facing the reality that I had a brain tumor waiting to be operated on in just a few hours.

OUR FINAL OUTING FROM THE hospital was to watch the Superbowl with Neil in our motel room. Jessica and I had shopped for fun deli food to make a buffet supper while we watched the game. As we left the hospital, we informed the on-duty nurse of what we were doing and where we were going. Although she wasn't keen on the idea, she made sure we had Neil's next dose of meds in hand. We hoped we wouldn't run into any of the doctors from Neurology on our way out the door.

We were beginning to feel a little uneasy, a little irresponsible, a little like law breakers. We were no longer the gregarious group of a few nights ago. We were tense and tight and tired.

Jackson had spent every night in the hospital, sleeping in the recliner by Neil's side. Mia was driving back and forth from her home an hour away, arranging time off from her nursing job in a hospital south of University-North, as well as trying to fit a few shifts in. She had come down with a bad cold and now Jim had caught it. Both were wearing surgical masks at our Superbowl gathering in order to protect Neil, but it cast a kind of gloomy pall on things.

We made our sandwiches and watched halfheartedly for a while, but Neil was disengaged and anxious and had had enough. He wanted to go back to the hospital and quit the charade. At half-time, he was back in his room.

~

The next day was the day before Neil's operation. It was a fairly uneventful day in the Waiting Game until early evening when all hell broke loose.

To pass the time and to calm our nerves we set out on a walk together—all of us. I don't know why, perhaps it was at the urging of the nurses, but we put Neil in a wheel chair with his dad pushing. Jessica, Jackson, Mia, and I made small talk as we took a familiar route toward the eclectic art exhibits that make University-North beautiful and impressive and add to the aura that this hospital is a place of healing.

We hadn't gone far when I looked up from a conversation I was having with Jessica and noticed Jim and Mia, their heads together, brows knit, looking as though they were trying to figure something out. In tandem, they turned around, swinging the wheelchair in a huge arc and started back toward the Neurology wing from where we had started just a few moments ago. Suddenly the leisurely walk became a hasty retreat, and I was taken completely by surprise.

"Something's wrong," Jim said. "We have to get Neil back to his room."

My mouth went dry and the prickly sound of fear filled my ears, drowning out everything around me.

"What's happening?" I asked, trying to keep up with them. "Neil, are you OK?"

He didn't answer me, just looked straight ahead, somewhat dazed and pale. Although I had no clarity of thought at that moment, I realize in hindsight that I was completely unprepared for anything but the Waiting Game that evening. That's what I knew, that's what I was bravely living through, that's what would morph into a different, unknown, and probably scary chapter tomorrow morning. But at least, on this last evening before my son had to endure brain surgery, I understood the plan, was holding my own emotionally, and felt confident that I could offer more strength than I really had to Neil before they wheeled him away from us to the operating room the next morning. But now everything seemed to be changing, and I couldn't understand.

Just as we were about to push the wheelchair into Neil's room he had a seizure; his body went limp with unconsciousness and at the same time, rigid with clenched muscles. His legs, which had been on the little perch of the wheelchair, shot out stiffly onto the floor, making it impossible to get him over the door jam into his room. As Jim and Mia struggled to maneuver, Neil came to, and along with Jackson they managed to get him into the room and onto his bed.

Then the room filled with people—several nurses, a couple of interns from Neurology, and all of us. After his brief regaining of consciousness, Neil began to seize again. Mia was up on the bed, holding him, Jim was on one side of him, and Jackson on the other. As he began to come to a second time, one of the interns also partially hoisted himself onto the bed and spoke to Neil, asking him to look at him and answer a question. Neil turned his head toward the intern's voice and said, "I can't see you. Oh, wait a minute, there you are...and a handsome fellow you are!"

Everyone in the room laughed. How could Neil still be so "Neil" while his vision malfunctioned and his body seized so violently? As he started to lose consciousness again, he said, "I feel like I am dying," and one of the nurses who had become so fond of him during the days leading up to this moment took his hand and said, "You are not dying—it only feels like it." She stayed by his side with her hand on his arm.

Something had to be done and fast. The decision was made to switch Neil to an alternate anti-seizure medication in an effort to stop the seizure activity before his scheduled surgery the next morning. Before it could be administered and take effect however, Neil had to live through this living hell again and again and we had to witness the shock of it all. Every time Neil regained consciousness, his eyes would search for and find his twin brother who was holding tight to his right hand. And this is an image permanently filed in the album of my mind even after eight years: Neil looking up with a beseeching look on his face, and Jackson returning his gaze with so much focus and so much love that it seemed as if a beam of light was passing back and forth between them.

And then I broke. Beside myself with shock and grief I was led out of the room just as the elevator opened and Jim's two sisters, Jane and Sali, stepped out. I greeted them with, "Neil is having seizures," and then had a sort of fit, crying again and again, "My baby, my baby, my baby, my baby." Somewhere inside me I think I recognized I was causing a disturbance, but who the hell cared—this was a hospital and nasty things must happen here all the time. My sisters-in-law led me down the hall and out of ear-shot of the pandemonium in Neil's room. They held me until I was able to calm down.

Worn out, empty, and eventually quiet, I retreated to a dark chamber inside myself that I never knew was there. And even though I may have looked the same on the outside, that's where I resided for the remainder of that horrible night.

*n*THE NEUROSURGEON WE FINALLY DECIDED on after days of uncertainty and feverish research was University-North's own Dr. Carrington. My entire family had met him and he instilled in us a confidence and a feeling of "rightness" that he was the one to undertake my intricate surgery.

The operation that was in store for me is called a craniotomy and my family was pleased that Dr. Carrington planned on using the latest technique, called brain mapping. Brain mapping involves using a probe with a low dose of electrical current to locate areas in the brain that govern the ability to speak or to move a part of the body. With the patient awake, or semi-awake, the surgeon can monitor his or her ability to perform these functions that could, potentially, be damaged. It allows the surgeon to remove the tumor to the maximum extent possible because of knowing which areas must be carefully navigated. The whole thing sounds macabre and unbelievable, but the fact is that the brain has no nerve endings, so pain is not an issue. And being awake and responsive, answering a question asked of me, would help Dr. Carrington locate more precisely the boundary between tumor and healthy brain matter.

The day before my surgery my family was suspended in two states simultaneously: relief that the day had finally arrived and unbelievable tension that the day had finally arrived. Anxiety was building hour by hour. Although we had made as much of a home in the hospital as we could, we were now like six hamsters crammed into a small cage. As evening set in, we needed a change of pace.

My mother suggested that we all take a last walk around the now too familiar hospital halls. As we let the nurse on duty know our plan, she asked that I be transported in a wheelchair for the outing and we agreed. Although it seemed unnecessary, I certainly wasn't offended by her request. It actually added some novelty to a mundane activity we'd done scores of time in the past five days. My dad started out pushing me, and Mia walked by my side. Despite the fears that each of us harbored inside, our mood switched from tight and tense to expansive and lighthearted. We were talking and laughing as if we were on a Sunday stroll with no troubles waiting down the road.

Then all of a sudden a strange feeling came over me—a change impossible to put into words. But I knew something wasn't right. Everything was sort of coming to a head, but I didn't know what "everything" was. I've been asked to describe a seizure by friends and family, but it's difficult. No matter what you are doing—having the time of your life, surrounded by loved ones, in the middle of laughing—all of a sudden, out of nowhere, you just know that something bad is about to happen. Before you've gained familiarity with plummeting into a seizure, you have no idea what's going on. Is the world about to end? Is everything supposed to be so dark? If this description leaves you feeling confused and not sure what I'm trying to convey, then that's the point. Because that is exactly what a seizure feels like. And then you just check out and lose all consciousness.

Needless to say, my wheelchair seizure the night before my scheduled operation scared the hell out of my whole family.

I regret that they had to witness it and the ones that followed. What I learned, after the fact, was that those seizures occurred like a string of firecrackers, flaring up and dying out before the next one ignited. I remember surfacing from a seizure a few times, feeling as though I was awakening from a bad dream and struggling to gain full consciousness. And I clearly recall thinking that what was happening to me was the process of dying.

Try as they did to control the seizure activity, nothing was effective. I was heavily sedated for the remainder of the night and, ultimately, lost my chance to participate in the brain mapping plan scheduled for the next morning. I don't dwell on it as there is no point crying over spilt milk. But it has crossed my mind, and why wouldn't it, that the life I got might have been different had I been able to stay conscious during my craniotomy.

*a*NEIL COULD NO LONGER STAY IN the big white room that had become all of ours. He had to be observed and monitored round the clock until early the next morning when Dr Carrington would open his skull and remove as much as he could of the tumor. Right across the hallway from his room was the intensive neurological unit, always brightly lit and ER-like, where patients in this more serious category needed to be. Neil was immediately moved into one of those beds.

There was nowhere to be with Neil in this new setting; he was sedated and it was now night time. Wearily, Jessica, Jackson, and Mia headed to the motel to get some rest. Jim and

I stayed behind. I perused the glaringly lit new setting with its multiple beds, central nursing station, and hard white floor. There was no obvious place for me here, no nook, no corner empty of hospital machines. I stood there with my pillow and blanket, scoping out how I could remain by Neil's side. Finally, all I could do was to drop my pillow on the floor as close to his bed as possible and curl up in my usual fashion. There was no way I was going to leave my baby.

After a moment or two, however, I realized that there was no place here for Jim. I had left him alone, standing somewhere on the outskirts. As this realization dawned on me, a beautiful young nurse who was in charge of this unit approached me. She spoke to me kindly, in no way demanding that I get up and leave my post. But her words made sense: "This floor is so hard and I don't want anyone to trip over you. Why don't you rest in the lounge down the hall, and I will get you if anything changes."

Having someone tell me what to do, to direct me, was exactly what I needed at this point. And I knew that Jim was suffering as much as I was. We needed to be together. The two of us made our way to the little lounge which, unlike it's appearance in daylight hours, was now dark and comfortingly cave-like. As we made our pallets side by side on the carpeted floor, we murmured hellos to the only other occupant in the room who would be our roommate for the night—a lovely woman wrapped in a blanket in a chair who was sitting vigil for her husband who was undergoing a similar crisis. Our hearts went out to each other, and our joint presence in the room that night was never an imposition or an issue.

And so began one of the most tortured nights of our lives. We slept some, changed the positions of our stiff bodies frequently, and were awake a good deal of the night. Sometime around dawn someone tapped my shoulder. I raised my bleary eyes to the beautiful young nurse, here to tell us that Neil was being prepped for surgery. The moment had arrived after countless hours of waiting.

"How is he?" I asked. " Did the seizures stop? Were you able to get them under control?"

Fully expecting that all had gone as planned with the new medication, she dealt me a terrible blow, despite the concern and sympathy for me I read in her eyes.

"No—nothing worked and we tried several different medications. He had seizures off and on all night long. We've been in touch with Dr. Carrington. The surgery will take place as scheduled, but it won't be possible to do the brain mapping with Neil awake and responsive. The doctor will have to perform the surgery with him fully sedated."

Jim and I rose from the floor, rumpled and heavy hearted. We were in agony for our son. He had endured days of having his life suspended, withstood unfathomable fear, had waited patiently for his brain mapping, his best chance of recovering from this terrible thing that had happened to him. He deserved his life back. He was a kind and decent person with so much life in him and so much life in front of him. Why did this have to happen?

And because we humans take life so personally, I railed

against the universe in those moments in that dark little waiting room. And then, of course, came the "what ifs." What if Neil could have had his operation just one day earlier, and WHY did he have to wait five f-ing days to get the help he needed immediately? Could I have done anything to change the course or the speed of things? And would I sink into craziness by playing these thoughts over and over, as if this was the only recording I owned?

As we folded our makeshift bedding in silence, we faced the plate glass window which looked out onto the hallway. And before our eyes appeared the beautiful nurse pushing a hospital gurney. And on the gurney, wrapped in a white sheet and cap, eyes closed and quiet, was our beloved son, unaware that his mom and dad were there, sending him our love and our blessings and wishing him godspeed. Once again, I had to deal with the unexpected and accept it. I never would have imagined that the Waiting Game would end this way. But that's how it played out.

FOUR

DARK DAYS

Some days I look down
Afraid I will fall
And though the sun shines
I see nothing at all
Then I hear your sweet voice
Oh, come and then go
Telling me softly
You love me so.

~ Patty Griffin

a WE LAID CLAIM TO SOME TERRITORY outside the operating rooms, like half a dozen other families that morning of February seventh. Jessica was not doing well. She was having trouble dealing with the stress we had endured the evening before and the vast unknown that lay before us. But being a therapist herself, she knew how to reach out for help. She had phoned her college friend, Amy, who lived not far from the medical center. Amy offered to leave her two little boys with her husband for a few hours and drive to the hospital to be with Jessica during Neil's surgery.

I left Jessica with Jim as she waited for her friend and went with Jackson and Mia to get something to eat. In the middle of our meal, Jessica, with Amy by her side, showed up at the doorway of the cafeteria. I got up to greet them, and Amy wrapped her arms around me. Her face was twisted with pain, and her eyes glistened with tears. As she separated from me, she held my shoulders, looked straight into my eyes and said, "You can do this." This dear friend, this gentle earth-mother, with her loving touch and her direct gaze injected some strength into me at that moment, re-instilling in me my long held belief that we function as angels for each other, and when we are sent forth, we aren't even aware of the job we are doing, the gift we just gave.

As I walked back to join Jim, I passed a couch and saw that Amy was sitting on one end of it, eyes closed, her body supported by its generous, cushioned arm. And Jessica was curled up against her, her head resting on her friend's shoulder. I knew my daughter was, literally, in good hands, and I breathed a prayer of thanks for the blessings amid despair—the tiny sprout that somehow can crack the sidewalk above it.

～

In our own ways we navigated the hours of Neil's surgery: we leafed through magazines, power-walked the hallways, did our best at everyday conversation, dozed off, and sat silently with our own private thoughts. At one point, Jim and I started off on yet another walk. We rounded the corner to the main lobby, and there on a couch in front of us were Jim's three siblings, his brother from Boston and his two sisters. We had not known they were there, sitting vigil apart from us but there for us in our hour of need. Their faces were strained, and I noticed that one of his sister's cheeks was tear stained. We hugged, let them know that we had no information yet; then suddenly, with no warning, Jim bolted from the group—just ran away, out of eye shot, down the hall from where we had emerged a moment earlier.

I bolted after him, calling, "Jim!" He had stopped, and as I caught up he broke into uncontrollable sobs. His body shook with all the pent up anguish he had been holding inside until the sight of his family broke him open. While I was becoming used to discharging my grief in public places, doing so was not Jim's style or within his comfort zone. So he'd simply had to remove himself. Before I could do or say anything to help him, he regained his composure—just like that, as though it had never even happened — and I was astounded at how he could do that and how differently we all exhibit our shock and grief.

After he rejoined his siblings in the lobby, my sisters-in-law suggested that we collect anyone who wanted to and go sit quietly in the chapel for a spell—spend some time in a quiet, peaceful atmosphere, designed to offer respite for those experiencing great suffering. While Jim, his brother, and Jackson decided to stay behind, our group of five women filed into the tiny, lovely chapel and sat in a row. Although I either gazed ahead at the altar or sat with my eyes closed, I could physically feel the presence of these familiar females, and I hoped beyond hope that the combined power of our prayers could beam its way into that operating room, fuse with the doctors' skills and my son's determination to live, and bolster the power of each.

With all the focus I could muster, I sent forth my prayer—"May all be well."

~

The hours passed and the time drew near for Neil's surgery to be completed, according to what we'd been told to expect. Jackson, Jessica, Mia, Jim, and I gathered at our station and waited. Before long Dr. Carrington emerged from the operating wing wearing his scrubs. As he walked toward us, I scrutinized him carefully for signs of distress: was his face pale, shut down, mask-like; were his shoulders sagging in defeat; did he look exhausted? To my hopeful relief, he looked pretty much as he had when we'd met him, youthful, despite his gray hair and glasses, erect and open-faced.

We followed him into a small consulting room. "How is Neil?" we asked. "How did the surgery go? How much of the tumor were you able to remove?" He told us that Neil was doing well and that he had been able to surgically remove about seventy percent of the tumor.

"His brain is now resting comfortably in his skull where it should be," he said. He told us that Neil was heavily sedated and in the Critical Care Unit. The sedation would slowly wear off, and by the end of the night or by the next morning, Neil could be moved back to the Neurology wing, and yes, we could see him at any point now, despite his being in a deep sleep.

Jim and the others were ready. I was not. I knew that I was living in a precarious emotional state, and I chose self-preservation above all else. It seems strange to me now. But at that time I was completely inexperienced with operations and hospitals and serious illness. My fear was stronger that I was. All I cared about was that Neil had made it through surgery, that that was behind him and he now could move on to the next step in this unwelcome journey.

When I heard from the others that Neil's face was extremely swollen and discolored on one side and he kind of didn't look like Neil, I felt I'd made the right decision for me. It would be one more day before I entered his room and took his hand. We all do what we can. I took heart and was satisfied with the knowledge that Neil was surrounded by bedside love from the other four. My love, on the other hand, had to float in with them, essence-like, and surround him like a vapor until I pulled myself together.

~

Dr. Carrington's prediction that Neil would be back in his room in Neurology in short order did not come to pass. A problem, which I guess could not be evaluated as Neil was transported, sedated, to Critical Care, was that he was unable to breathe on his own. This involuntary function had become temporarily paralyzed as a result of the surgery. When the Respiratory Specialist in Critical Care attempted to remove Neil's breathing tube, he began to choke and had to be reintubated immediately. Given this situation, Neil had to remain sedated while a machine performed the task that he was unable to do on his own.

Dr. Carrington, while not expecting this, was not surprised either. He assured us that this happens sometimes after brain surgery. In some cases it can take a day or two for the patient to resume the involuntary functions, but it would happen. And so we rested assured. They would try again in a day or two to remove the tube, at which point Neil would undoubtedly be more stable, more healed, and ready to bid farewell to Critical Care. I remember thinking to myself how unfair it was to be suspended in yet another waiting game, but a day or two would be a pittance in comparison to the week we had just endured.

And so we took up a new residency within the hospital in the Critical Care Waiting Room, a darkened, den-like, sheltered-from-the-public enclave where families gathered with whatever would make them comfortable—knitting, cross-words, cards, games, reading material—as they waited word on their loved ones across the hall in Critical Care. The room was lined with comfortable chairs, but the most sought after, the ones families made a bee-line to and arrived early to nab, were the recliners. Folks would set up little tent cities on and surrounding their recliners, furnished with blankets and pillows stored in the roomy closet for anyone to borrow. The recliners were great to nap in.

The Critical Care Waiting Room was its own little country within the borders of the larger hospital. If you happened to be a citizen there, you felt well cared for, you felt empathy for your neighbors, but each and every citizen was hoping to defect as soon as possible. Some were able to do just that. Their loved ones were coming out of anesthesia following surgery and doing what their doctors expected—progressing as anticipated. Other citizens had to wait longer for their walking papers and became familiar faces, "elders," in this tense, uncertain society. At the helm was the Critical Care Waiting Room attendant who manned the phone at the front desk. I think the hospital must have selected its nicest, most caring and sincere employees for this job, for every attendant was warm, patient, and gracious. They would relay calls from the CCU to those of us camped out and waiting for progress reports from doctors.

There was also a direct phone line for family members to use, as we could not enter Critical Care without asking permission. It became a regular routine each morning for us to pick up the phone and ask whoever answered in CCU if we could come in. They would check, usually say, "Yes, come on in," or sometimes, "Wait ten minutes until we've completed our morning routine with Neil." And that's how it all worked.

Being a citizen of the CCU society was a little like residing in Hades. It certainly was better than Hell—we knew that because we'd already had a glimpse of that frightful place. In Hades, you hoped that you'd get a second chance, that because you were a basically good person and tried hard to be patient, you might get moved to a slightly nicer place. That's what we were aiming for and had our hearts set on.

~

Dr. Carrington sent the respiratory specialist to remove Neil's breathing tube for the second time. The procedure involved taking Neil off sedation and asking him to wake up and participate to the best of his ability. Jim and Jessica were present as Neil's coaches and advocates. As he began to gain some consciousness and move around, they spoke to him, telling him they were there and asking him to stay present.

The removal of the tube causes the body to react exactly the way it's portrayed on all of the TV hospital shows. The patient gags and coughs violently, and the body lunges and recoils involuntarily. It's not pretty. While everyone present was hoping for the best, was rooting him on, the result of this second attempt was complete failure. It was not that Neil was unable to breathe on his own due to an issue with his lungs. The problem was that the continued paralysis of his throat made it impossible for him to swallow his saliva. Mucous would collect and he would begin to choke. The tube had to go back in, and Neil had to resume his drugged sleep. It was a total bummer. We were going nowhere fast.

And so began another dip into Hell with all the unknowns and grim outlooks and nasty twists and turns. While Dr. Carrington understood our concern and frustration, he wanted to give Neil more time to heal. If, after the third try, Neil still could not swallow and, therefore, breathe on his own, he would insert a tracheotomy so that Neil could at least be allowed to come back into a conscious state and move from the CCU. Only then, we knew, could we really assess our son's condition.

The days dragged on. Neil's dear friend, Seth, who was living in Aspen, Colorado, flew in to sit by Neil's bedside just to be there for him. Seth would return to his mom's home in northern Vermont each night and return to keep vigil the next day. I was touched by Seth's love and his loyalty, but I had nothing in me to even try to connect and show my gratitude to him, to ask him about his life or make the simplest pleasantry. I knew that Seth understood and would never want me to give more than I could, but it felt weird to just nod my head to him in passing, this dear boy who was special to all of us. But that's just the way it was. I would tell Neil about the time Seth spent by his side much later. He never knew his friend had been there for him—in body as well as spirit.

And there were a few other visitors who came to buoy us up as best they could. With the exception of Seth, I did not allow anyone but family members to see Neil in such a horribly diminished state. Later, I heard that Mia took extreme exception to this, but that was my position and I stood by it. Neil was surrounded by his closest loved ones for most of every day. He didn't need to be the comatose center of attention for others.

One afternoon I was sitting by Neil's side in the CCU. He had been on his back for so long that the nurses had decided to arrange him in an upright, sitting position, out of his bed, in a special chair. I looked up at him. He seemed suspended so high, his eyes were closed, and his head was bent forward. He still wore the little post-surgical cap that covered his scar. It struck me suddenly, and with deep sorrow, that in this never ending state of sleep he had been reduced to a mere object. He was the center of my attention but he was completely inanimate.

Just then, the middle aged parents of one of Neil's friends entered the room. The mother had been a nurse herself, knew the ins and out of hospital life, had had the CCU Waiting Room attendant call in and ask for permission to enter, had been granted permission and had, bold as brass, done so.

What nerve! As soon as I recovered from the shock of seeing them in my baby's room, I yelled, "Get Out! You can't be in here!" and they beat a hasty retreat, probably wondering what my problem was. I know they were just trying to show their concern, their support. But to me it was a boundary-issue intrusion.

On the flip side, a colleague of Jim's, together with her husband, drove the hour and fifteen minutes north to the hospital just to drop off a beautiful basket of sweets and grapes with a card telling us we were in their hearts. They left their gift at the front desk and turned around and drove all the way back. Their gesture astounded us.

Many notes, cards and letters arrived each day. Some of Neil's cousins sent memories of their early lives together. My tennis friends sent money. Parents of Neil's students wrote. Members of our community who were not among our closest friends took the time to tell us that we were in their thoughts and prayers, conveying the message that we are all in this boat named "Life" together, we are all human and can acknowledge, with compassion, the difficulties in each other's lives. These kindnesses had a profound impact on me. I vowed never to procrastinate on reaching out to others to simply say, "I know you are in pain, and I am thinking of you."

A friend of Jessica's whom Jim and I had never met dropped off a small white board and marker so that when he was ready, Neil could write what he wanted to say if he was not yet ready to use his voice due to his airway problems. And Judy took over all communications between us and the outside world, canceled our airline tickets to Florida, and even accompanied me to my doctor to secure the paperwork for a medical leave of absence from my job. Given the fact that many times a day I would just stare off into space, be functional but not really "all there," I knew I was not able to resume my teaching responsibilities. Judy and I sat in the doctor's office with our arms around each other and cried through the whole appointment together. My dear, dear comrade through this roller coaster of life.

∼

Talking about psychic pain in her writings, author Sylvia Boorstein says that because change is the nature of existence, sometimes a window will open briefly during a particularly anguished time, and we are released from pain's headlock. It's a little vacation, a little gift, a little miracle. Jessica and I had such an experience. We climbed out of the darkness one evening at our home in the Days Inn.

Earlier that day, a friend from out of state, who happened to be in Vermont on business, came by the hospital to give us hugs and moral support. Our friend is very "New Age-y" and spiritually oriented. After hugging us good-bye, she put her hands over her heart, and her face took on a kind of far-away, winsome, "I hold you in my heart" look. There is no doubt that her visit had been good for us, had given us diversion from the long, stressful hours. What we didn't realize was that it was a gift that kept on giving.

That night in our room, as we were eating, I turned to Jessica, put my hands over my heart and made "the face." Jessica burst out laughing. She did it back to me and I lost it. And the next minute we were flopping on the bed and rolling on the floor in uncontrollable laughter. We were in hysterics. All we had to do at that point was look at each other, and the laughter would explode all over again. When this fit finally subsided, our bellies ached, our cheeks were wet, our clothes were rumpled, our hair disheveled, but we felt better. We had been transported out of our shriveled, miserable selves to a place of lightness. We humans are such a strange and complex package. And thank you dear friend, for lifting us into the light. We want you always in our lives.

$\sim$

Meanwhile, things with Neil were very bad. And not just bad in a "state-of-suspension" kind of way. Every day brought more grim news, additional problems and downturns which were always unforeseen and left us barely able to keep our balance. Dr. Carrington had already told us that Neil's tumor proved to be a stage three malignancy. He had referred Neil's case to the highly-regarded neurological oncologist, Dr. Marcel Renaud. Dr. Carrington told us that our hospital was very lucky to have and to hold onto someone of Dr. Renaud's caliber and that he, himself, would, in a heartbeat, send any of his family members to be patients of Renaud if they needed treatment for brain cancer. We would meet Dr. Renaud in a few days time after the oncologist looked in on Neil and did an initial assessment, despite the fact that Neil was still "under."

Although I wished that Neil's diagnosis had been better, I was not surprised. I mean what were the chances that this thing was benign? I had never hung my hat on that hope. And at least stage three was better than stage four. I had to take my solace where I could. But there was more. Dr. Carrington told us that "it could be nothing," but Neil's latest MRI revealed some areas in the brain that looked as if small strokes had occurred. They could have been the result of the many uncontrollable seizures the night before his surgery.

I felt a rage rising within me. And then, perhaps because of the numbness which now superseded any other emotion, it ceased to roil. There was simply no place to hold it. Where could I even go with this information? I looked evenly at Dr. Carrington while I felt that warm fog, like a protective blanket, wrap itself around my mind, shielding me from a lethal case of the same "what ifs" I'd experienced after our horrific night on the floor of the neurological oncology waiting room. I chose to focus solely on the "it could be nothing." My team needed me, and I needed to stay upright despite blows coming from all directions.

Deflecting blows became our whole life now. Due to lying comatose for days, Neil had developed blood clots in both arms. His upper arms were gigantic and looked like two beached whales. It upset me to look at them. Due to the fact that it was obvious that he had clots in his arms, the doctors did a sonogram of his lower body and found, unsurprisingly, that he had a clot in one of his legs as well.

A blood clot in the leg can be dangerous. If it dislodges and makes its way through an artery to the heart or lung, the situation could be fatal. A standard protective measure is to insert a little barrier screen called a shunt into the main artery of the leg to keep this hazardous journey from occurring. And so it happened that Neil had to be transported from the CCU to another operating room where this procedure took place.

Our hope was that the blood thinner that Neil was being administered intravenously would dissolve the blood clots in his arms. However, upon arriving at his bedside a day or two later, we found that his whole upper body had broken out in a spotty red rash. Neil was allergic to the blood thinner and had to be taken off of it and put on an alternative medication.

It felt as though there was never a morning that held any improvement, any hope, any light. These beginning of the day visits took a terrible emotional toll on us, individually and as a couple. We aimed to be present in the CCU when the team of doctors and medical students made their morning rounds. We wanted information, to share our own observations, and to ask questions.

Jim and I, like plenty of couples, have different styles of conducting ourselves, especially under stress. He is generally calm, organized, direct, soft spoken, and polite, with his questions well thought out. I am also direct and courteous but a little intense. More than once, Jim felt that I was bringing up questions that had been covered and addressed. I could see that we were getting in each other's way. I felt that he was put on edge by my morning contributions and realized that he was doing his own best job of holding it together under incredible stress. And I knew that he was trying to protect me. It got to the point that when the team appeared at our door, Jim would suggest that he speak to the doctors by himself as Neil's condition was so difficult for me to deal with. Jim and I were team members, yet I understood that we all have our roles, and that I might not be the most effective participant for the morning conference. I accepted that and stepped out of the way. He could fill me in later. It worked for me.

∼

The first room that Neil had been moved to in the CCU directly following his surgery was worse than awful. It didn't actually feel like a room. It was more like a brightly lit cubical with a wider than usual door that everyone who entered or exited the CCU had to walk past. We hated everything about it: the constant noise, its lack of privacy, its size, and the fact that it had no windows. We could see that there were other much nicer rooms in this unit which were larger, more private, and had sunny windows facing the New Hampshire woods. But they were all occupied and Neil was the newcomer. All we could hope was that one of the better rooms would open up and Neil could be moved.

In keeping with the downward spiral of things, another issue emerged which we had to deal with as best we could: Neil displayed a form of agitation during nighttime hours which is common to patients who are suspended in intensive care units. Neil's agitation manifested in his continual attempts to pull out his breathing tube. He had managed to accomplish this several times. It was of concern to the nighttime staff as the consequences could be dire if he was not caught and stopped. It wasn't possible to assign one attendant to any one patient so it was decided to encase Neil's hands in large, thick bed mittens.

As Jim and I would prepare to take our leave of the hospital and return to Day's Inn, the night shift would be arriving. If the nurse in charge of Neil was one I knew and liked, who was personally invested in Neil's well being, then I could leave in peace. If a new nurse arrived, or a nurse I felt did not meet the necessary qualifications, I was unsettled and unhappy, and I would want to linger to make sure we were all on the same page regarding Neil's care. Hard as it was to leave Jim would pull me away for my own good. I never left, however, until those mittens were solidly in place.

The mittens worked well for a time, but, eventually, Neil figured out how to clap both mittened hands together to dislodge the tube. At that point, there was no option but to restrain his arms for the night in an effort to protect him.

n "I AM AWAKE—AT LEAST I THINK I AM. But where am I? In a bed, but not my own. Is this a dream? Because all kinds of contraptions are working against me. Strings or hoses are attached to my arms. I want to rub my eyes out of their sleepy state but I can't pull my arm up. Both of my hands are tied down. What the hell is going on? I think my hands are zipped into some sort of pillow cases. Have I gone insane? Why else would I be tied to the bed like a crazy person?"

I start to panic and writhe against my hindrances. Why won't anyone help me? From a distance, I hear my father's voice. I know it's my dad, though I cannot locate him: "Neil—stop —leave it alone. No, Neil." And then he is gone, and I am gone too.

Being in the heavily sedated state I was suspended in during that time—days that were interminable for my family and mostly non-existent for me —I have no memory of pulling my breathing tube out. Pieces of those days are scattered around my mind like a thousand piece jigsaw puzzle dumped out on the floor. I know I'll never be able to assemble the pieces to form the whole picture. Now and then a memory, a piece of the puzzle, will be revealed out of nowhere. Maybe I smell something or feel something that somehow kicks my memory into turbo mode, and I get the sense of deja vu. And then again, the writing of this sorry part of my life is like a prompt that calls back a missing piece.

Later on, I learn second-hand about my blood clots, my allergies to the meds I was receiving, my inability to breathe on my own, and the squawking alarm that was eventually attached to my gown to alert the nursing staff of my attempts to exit the bed, but I have virtually no solid memories of my ICU days and I am grateful for that. I was, however, vaguely conscious of the coming and going of doctors and nurses and the presence of my family—their disembodied voices. I knew that I was not completely alone.

a JACKSON HAD RETURNED TO HIS JOB in New York City. He, like his father, kept his emotions stowed away inside, but I knew how vulnerable he was with his twin brother in such a precarious state up in New England. I was grateful he had Sarah, his girlfriend, now his wife, by his side. He had love and support and someone with whom he could share his grief. Jessica was back in North Carolina without the same kind of support, and I knew she was in a fragile state. Unlike Jackson, she could not just hop in the car on the weekend to rejoin us in New Hampshire. I hoped that her job and colleagues offered some escape from her worries, but I knew we were almost constantly on her mind.

And so it was that just three of us, Jim, Mia, and I, met Dr. Renaud, the neurological oncologist assigned to Neil, for the first time. Karen Robinson, the hospital social worker who had been so helpful to Neil, informed us that Dr. Renaud was ready to confer with our family and had asked that we gather in the CCU Waiting Room prior to our meeting.

As we sat among others, a short, fit, balding man, with

beautiful posture and a presence both gentle and commanding, entered the room and made his way around, checking in with other patients' families. Mia told me that this was Dr. Renaud. He had been pointed out to her earlier that week. Karen entered the room, rounded us up, and ushered us into a small conference room so we could meet with Dr. Renaud in private. I imagine myself being anxious and tense before the meeting, though thinking back now, I don't recall any pre-meeting feelings at all. I just did what I was told, showed up when and where I was expected.

Dr. Renaud entered the small, windowless room and pulled a chair up, forming a little circle with Jim, Mia, Karen Robinson, and me. I remember thinking how accessible and informal Dr. Renaud's style was. He wasn't delivering his message behind an imposing desk. He just sat down with us, close and personal.

He told us, in much more detail than I can recount, that Neil's tumor consisted of two different types of malignancies and, therefore, was a "mixed" breed. It was called Oleoden-droglioma, and it was, unfortunately, incurable. In addition, if there can BE any addition to news like this, he told us that upon examining Neil, it appeared as though his mouth and his face on the right side were paralyzed (something I had not noticed due to Neil's airway tube prohibiting the possibility of speech or movement) and that he had weakness on the right side of his body in general. He said he knew that Neil had been a teacher and an athlete, and although it's possible I misinter-preted his message, it seemed to infer that upon his release from the hospital, Neil should try to live the best life possible, but it would not be the life that he had had.

I felt lightheaded as I tried to grasp what Dr. Renaud was saying. But my mind could contain only so much. It seemed to have erected a fortress of stone designed to keep horrors out and to protect the fragile me within. What were the ramifications of this doctor's message, the future results of what they had found embedded in Neil? Unspoken words such as "diminished" and "limited" regarding Neil's future life and "hopeless" regarding any future at all began to erode those walls of defense. Was this coming from me, my own dizzy mind, or was this what I was meant to take away?

I was not able nor did I want to ask him any questions. Our lives had just been crushed, pulverized. What was the point in saying, "Could you please be more specific? And could you give us a prognosis on his cognitive functioning?" What was the point in asking for more pain than had just been delivered? We had, in my mind, just been issued a death sentence.

The three of us sat there immobilized, saying nothing, not responding in any way. And I could feel that our stony silence had the effect of a dismissal of Dr. Renaud and Karen Robinson from our presence. It was not appropriate that they should even be with us now, and I felt that the three of us were one person in wanting them GONE. The claustrophobic air in that tiny, horrid room became charged with our need to be alone, our retreat from further discourse. Dr. Renaud rose, along with Karen, and silently left the room. We knew that we would meet with him again in a few days time to receive more specific test results and to discuss the next steps in Neil's treatment.

The second the door shut we collapsed. The three of us sobbed and sobbed. We were absolutely beside ourselves with shock and grief and disbelief. We held each other, and our bodies shook until we were weak. Mia kept crying over and over, "We were just beginning our life together." Seeing her beautiful tear-streaked face, distorted in agony, made my heart break open for her and for the future that was being ripped away from her. Hadn't she already had more than her share of troubles in her life? Why was this happening to our Neil and to us as a family, and why was the situation always so extreme and so dire? Why was it such, in this whole nightmarish journey, that we could never ever catch a break? It was all too unreal. Too devastating and unreal.

∾

Lesley and Kimberley, my sisters from Connecticut, were driving to New Hampshire to bring us a home-cooked meal the very afternoon of the meeting with Dr. Renaud. Our families now had a phone tree. We would call someone daily, and they, in turn, would start the communication chain to keep everyone in the loop and to save us from having to repeat our woes more than once. It often brought me pain to think of the pain our families were in. We are from close knit clans, and a member's troubles affected everyone. My sisters had booked a room at the Days Inn and had arranged to borrow some extra chairs and one of the tables from the lobby to turn their room into as fancy a dining space as they could, complete with tablecloth, candles, flowers and wine. They were on their way, and the fact that Jim and Mia and I were completely depleted from our hysterical meltdown could not change our plans.

The trip north went more quickly than my sisters anticipated. They had checked into Days Inn, gotten organized, and rather than waiting for us to arrive at our arranged time, they drove the few miles to the hospital to meet us there and to see the setting where we spent our days.

The main mall of University-North has a striking three story glass ceiling, and you can always tell the weather or what time of day it is by walking or sitting in the mall. During prime office and visiting hours, basically every day, five days a week, it is busy and energetic in a city-type way. It's an interesting place to people-watch. At night and on the weekends, however, it becomes quiet and lifeless, and the hours go by very slowly.

After pulling ourselves together as best we could, Jim and Mia and I left the little room attached to the CCU waiting room and prepared to gather our things to return to the motel. I must have needed to clear my head by taking a walk away from the CCU and the horror that had just occurred there, for I can see myself walking back through the mall, now nearly empty of pedestrians, to pick up my belongings and there, in the semi-darkness of that late February afternoon, looking down at me from the balcony of the CCU, one story up from the mall, were my sisters, come to find me. They descended the stairs, and as they walked toward me I began to cry.

Without saying anything they put down their purses and wrapped their arms around me in a tight three-way hug. As I melted into their supportive bodies, I relayed the devastating facts from the meeting with Dr. Renaud. As we held onto each other and rhythmically swayed, they offered me a different perspective and one they stated with conviction: that it was totally possible for Neil to get better, and they felt strongly that he would. Doctors always have to present the worst scenarios, and then patients get busy with the job their bodies are meant to do: heal.

The evening my sisters put on was just what we needed. Once again, we were lifted into the light of the outside world with new energy, hope, chit-chat conversation, good food, even laughter. I know my sisters must have been very upset and not prepared for what had come their way. But they came to do a job, and they did it well. They infused us with the strength we needed to get up the next morning and carry on.

~

A day or two later I ran into Karen Robinson in the hall by chance. We stopped to talk; she asked how I was doing, and she brought up our meeting and how she and Dr. Renaud had intuited that we wanted to be left alone. I told her how we had broken down and had been left feeling completely hopeless and bereft.

She felt bad about the scene I portrayed of Jim, Mia, and me beside ourselves with grief, of our being left so utterly destroyed. Yes, it was true that tumors such as these had the tendency to grow back, but amid the shock and fear that families feel receiving such news, most ask, "So what can you do for me, what is the next step, what is the recommended course of treatment?" There always are next, positive, proactive, hopeful steps—a plan.

I realized then and there in that hallway that Karen's words were not rehearsed, planned in advance, carefully crafted, just for me. She didn't know she would be seeing me. What she said was spontaneous, based on knowledge and experience. What she offered was not much, but it was something.

"I'm not naturally a very brave person," I confessed. I can hear myself saying those exact words to her as we stood there, though I don't recall in what context this admission was offered. But there it was —the secret belief I'd harbored all my life. Karen's eyes welled up. She looked directly into my eyes and her voice was firm despite the emotion I could read on her face: "I think you are a very brave person."

As I walked away a new knowledge germinated deep within me. Maybe, probably, I was not naturally brave. There was no shame in that. But people, mothers, human beings become brave when there is no choice in the matter. There are circumstances in life that bring on the spontaneous rising of qualities that you don't recognize as being "you." We are capable of surprising even ourselves.

~

Despite this conversation and the possibility of a different perspective, Jim and I had to face the fact that our son had been diagnosed with a large, "incurable," malignant brain tumor, seventy percent of which had been surgically removed and thirty percent which remained. If its nature was to sprout again and again despite attempts to cut it out with a scalpel and zap it with radiation and poison it with chemotherapy, what was the point? Why should Neil endure cruel treatments that would undermine the quality of his young life without the possibility of ever regaining a good life, or life at all? Without doing a lot of processing together—we pretty much kept our own counsel during these few days —we had come to the same position. We wanted, as soon as possible, to take our boy home with us to Westminster West where he had grown up, far away from this unhappy, unfamiliar place, to live as great a life as he could for as long as he had. And that is what we told Dr. Renaud on the occasion of our second meeting.

But Dr. Renaud cut us off. He had no intention of hearing us out. He had plans of his own to outline. "No, no, no," he insisted. "I have just received the report from the Mayo Clinic. The biopsy contains a genetic marker indicating that this tumor is very receptive to treatment with Temodar, the most effective drug for Neil's type of brain tumor. This is good news. The standard treatment today is six weeks of radiation to the brain followed by a one year course of the chemotherapy drug. I have made an appointment for you with Dr. Rider from radiology to learn more and to make a treatment decision. Radiation to the brain might have some troubling effects which can show up later in life. The decision is yours to make regarding taking the Temodar alone or in conjunction with radiation. The decision does not have to be made immediately. But you must learn about and consider all your options."

I was beginning to think that for us Taylors the tables don't just "turn;" they spin in a dizzy, disorienting way. We were not used to anything resembling good news or positive progress coming our way. We certainly did not expect this second meeting with Dr. Renaud to be in any way different from our first encounter. Why would it be? The orbit of our life had become an emotional roller coaster ride of anxious, dread-filled ups and sickening, downhill plunges. But here, in Dr. Renaud's office, we experienced some even ground, and for the first time in too long, we gained a measure of relief and hope.

∼

Dr. Rider, the radiologist, had an easy-going, direct manner. He also had strong opinions regarding the best course of action. He explained that in dealing with brain tumors such as Neil's, the double treatment of radiation followed by chemotherapy was the "thorough" standard. "And why wouldn't anyone want to throw the whole kitchen sink at this thing?" he asked. We all acknowledged that Neil had youth and increasing strength on his side. If he had to live with some negative side effects as an older person, he could deal with them then. Dr. Rider's conviction was just what we needed and, grateful for his direction, we signed up for the whole kitchen sink.

Learning that there was a recommended, appropriate

course of treatment for Neil shifted my thinking without my being aware that it was happening or that it had happened. Here is how I discovered it. Jim and I had left the hospital for a mental-health break to grab a beer and lunch at a nearby Irish pub. As we waited for our food, I began recounting all that I remembered from our second meeting with Dr. Renaud and the course of treatment that lay ahead of us. Jim seemed quiet, listening to me verbalize about the future. And then he said, "You have to remember that a treatment doesn't neces-sarily mean a cure. Neil may not be able to recover from this." And out of my mouth flew a response, calm, firm, direct and "knowing" —"I don't believe that for a second!"

I recognized that something strange had just occurred. Right after my response I thought to myself, "Where did that come from?" Because it came without considering or reflecting or choosing to disagree. It seemed to come from a place outside of me; I was merely the channel. The words had great power but no "feeling" quality to them. I didn't feel happy or relieved or that I needed to defend my position in any way. I just had a simple conviction.

*n*AWAKE AGAIN. IT'S SO INCREDIBLY DARK—it must be the middle of the night. I stretch my neck from side to side, searching for something familiar, something to give me a clue about where I am. I blink my eyes to focus on some form that might help me. Is there a digital alarm clock, an illuminated EXIT sign—anything I can spot in order to orient myself? For some reason, nothing comes into focus. When is it ever this dark, so black you can't see anything with your eyes wide open?

I remember this kind of night at Camp Takota when Jackson and I were very young. I remember being spooked then too by the all-pervasive darkness in those old cabins. I know I'm not at Camp Takota, and I know for sure that Jackson isn't here in the bunk below me. But the blackness is just the same.

I have to get out of this bed. I have to investigate, to figure out if I'm trapped inside a bad dream or whether this is real. Wait...I think I am in a hospital; I remember that smell. I twist my body sideways. I will my legs to follow but they feel heavy and separate from me. I push hard and I fall. I taste blood as my tooth sinks into my tongue. But then the blackness of unconsciousness descends, like always.

a WHEN WE RETURNED FROM OUR outing, one of the nurses approached us and informed us, apologetically, that while we were gone, Neil had attempted to get up and, in the process, had fallen out of bed. What could we say? What had happened had happened and was done with. But it probably wasn't a good thing for a guy who had recently undergone brain surgery to have taken a possible header on the hospital floor.

Directly following this incident the staff decided to move Neil's bed in the direct sight line of the nursing station, and to clip a portable alarm to his hospital gown which was programmed to go off if he moved too aggressively.

∾

Neil was becoming a long-term resident of the CCU. He still spent most of the day in a semi-sedated sleep and received all medications and nourishment through a central line attached to his arm. At 225 pounds on his six feet two inch frame, he had entered the hospital at his highest ever weight. Now he had lost fifty pounds. Mia was greatly concerned with this quick downward spiral. I had not liked the fact that Neil had let himself get overweight, but I certainly could understand that losing this much weight in a matter of weeks was extreme. When I looked at Neil's arms and legs, it was obvious that he was losing muscle. Because of Neil's inactive state, and because he exhibited weakness on his right side, the hospital physical therapists began working with him several times a week.

They were wonderful. The moment they entered the room they spoke cheerfully to Neil, always treating him like an active participant, despite the fact that he was more like a sleepy rag doll. They manipulated his arms and legs, wrists and ankles. Jim watched them carefully, asked questions, and completely took over the exercise regime on the days the PTs were not assigned to come, as well as on weekends when very few services were available to patients. Jim had always worked out and lifted weights with his two body-building sons and had a comfortable, confident working knowledge of body mechanics. He was used to the practice of pushing oneself, going for one more rep, one more pump. The guys in our household were committed to exercise, to the discipline it required, and the accompanying sense of accomplishment it yielded. They thrived on the camaraderie of working out together as well as the endorphin-fueled sense of well-being that followed. And so it was just natural that Jim became Neil's number one trainer and coach. As he worked Neil's limbs, Jim focused on the weaker right side, entreating Neil to squeeze, push, lift, flex, resist. And Neil responded to all commands. Sometimes his squeeze was more like a flutter, his flex just a tiny twitch. But a deep contentment settled over me during these sessions. My guys were working out together once again.

*IN A RAGDOLL STATE OF MIND, submerged in a world of total darkness, I began the uphill journey of rehabilitation. At the start, I was still semi-conscious and flat on my back in my hospital bed. I was pulled into awareness by people stretching out my legs and feet. And then they would start on my arms and hands. I had no strength at all. In all the weeks that had passed I hadn't even sat up on my own. Now, during my increasing periods of consciousness, I began to explore my body. I touched my arms, my chest, my head. I was shocked. I didn't recognize myself. Even my head didn't feel familiar. It felt like a misshaped skull with an enormous indented scar still covered by thick scab. My arms felt like Mia's arms, narrow and feminine—nothing like my own. My chest was frail and meatless. Gone were the pectoral muscles that I had worked so hard to develop. In my mind I looked emaciated, a replica of third world citizens from war-torn lands that had shocked me as a child pouring over issues of National Geographic. Like them, I had lost muscle as well as fat.

This new knowledge of my physical self was revealed by my tactile sense, alone. Why could I still see nothing? Why were my eyes not working? I needed to ask this question—to shout it out as loud as I could—though that was not possible. All that was left of me and left to me were my questions, swirling around endlessly, nearly driving me crazy.

THE FACT THAT NEIL WAS RESPONDING to the PTs and Jim's commands was very gratifying. He could hear us, could understand, and could respond. And he displayed motivation. All good signs. Even before the PT workouts, very soon after his surgery, we would stand by his bedside and ask him simple questions that required simple responses: "Do you have a dog?" "Do you love us?" —dumb stuff like that, to which he would slowly nod his head. It brought us a measure of hope and gratitude.

We realized before we got too far with this game, however, that the questions we presented were ones which would elicit a positive response from Neil—a head nod. Jessica had come for a weekend visit and was reporting Neil's progress to her childhood friend Abby one evening during this period, and they began brainstorming questions to which Neil would most likely respond in the negative if he was in full charge of his faculties, if he was the Neil we knew before undergoing brain surgery. According to Jessica, Abby proclaimed, "I've got it! Ask him if he likes George Bush!"

Next morning, as soon as she was admitted to the CCU, Jessica leaned over Neil's hospital bed and asked, "Neil, I have a question for you. Do you like George Bush?"

There was no gap, no hesitation on Neil's part. He slowly but clearly and firmly shook his head back and forth from side to side. The Neil we knew was still among us.

*n*IN MY LUCID MOMENTS, WHEN MY consciousness would rise to the surface for a spell, I became aware that my family was asking questions. This was different from the murmurs of love and encouragement that helped soothe me in the past. It began to dawn on me that the questions were for me. I'm sure I was foggy from sedatives, but the George Bush question was like shooting fish in a barrel. I shook my head from side to side in what I now envision as a "Hell No" response—proof that I could truly understand what was being asked of me. That part of my brain still worked. And somehow it dawned on me that this simple reaction was, to my family, a small but significant gift.

*a*NEIL'S PERIODS OF CONSCIOUSNESS BEGAN to

increase as the days went by. The immediate goal before him was to sleep less and be awake for longer stretches each day. However, the physical trauma of having one's skull peeled back and brain rearranged demands major healing time, and there is no greater agent of healing than sleep. We may have wanted "more," but Neil's body had its own intelligence.

One afternoon I happened to be standing, looking out the window of the CCU waiting room, facing the doors of the CCU. I watched the door swing open, and Jim and Mia walked through, laughing and talking to each other with great animation. I walked out to greet them, and they told me excitedly that Neil had seemed sufficiently awake for them to place the white board that we had received as a gift into his left hand and the marker into his weak right hand. They told him to try and write the answer to their question. They asked him, "Neil—do you know where you are?" and in wispy, wobbly letters, somewhat piled up on each other he wrote, "hospital." They showed me the whiteboard, proof that, cognitively, Neil was capable of more than "yes" and "no" responses. We hugged each other in celebration of this small but significant step. And, further, it was not insignificant to me that the word "hospital" was spelled correctly!

I REMEMBER THE LITTLE WHITEBOARD. At first, trying to write was next to impossible. Not only was I weak from being sedated and tied down for so long, but I was suffering from partial paralysis on the right side of my body. Nevertheless, I wanted to communicate, to feel connected, to express myself. The white board became my mode of communication, my only tool for several weeks.

Initially it was a challenge to even grasp the marker and try to control its movement, but one day, while I was still in the CCU, my father asked me, "Neil, do you know where you are?" I knew by then, of course I did. He put the marker in my feeble right hand and the board in my steadier, normally-functioning left hand. Doing the best I could, I slowly, carefully, spelled out h-o-s-p-i-t-a-l across the smooth surface of the whiteboard. Mia hugged me and my dad laughed and teased me about my lackluster penmanship. Somehow it dawned on me that they had just given me another test, and in those few moments I gave back evidence that I was capable of answering a question with more that just a head shake or nod. I could actually form a word in response. For a moment, their happiness was mine. But that moment was short lived.

I began to realize during this dreamlike time of my life that my eyes were not working. I couldn't see anything. Every time I was conscious I would attempt to look around and get my bearings, but it was as though I hadn't even opened my eyes. I was living in total darkness. The only joy I felt during this confusing and frightening period was my growing awareness that my loved ones, my immediate family and Mia, were at my bedside. They were with me. I could pick out the voices of my mother, my father, Mia, Jackson, Jessica, and they helped me feel less alone and separated from life. Deep within, I knew that they were going through this terrible ordeal with me. They had never left me.

Despite the gratifying progress I was making in using the white board to communicate responses to my family, not all my simple messages brought them happiness. I penned one that broke my mother's heart. She told me about it later when we were finally able to communicate verbally and it breaks my own heart to think about it. She came into my room one morning and picked the board up from my lap. I had worked on my message long before anyone had arrived. It contained seven simple words, the longest of which had a mere four letters: "I cant see I am so sad."

a I WAS OFTEN PRESENT IN NEIL'S room in the CCU when it was time for the attending nurse to do a check of his vital signs and automatic responses. He or she would go through the routine, including opening his eyelids and shining a flashlight into his eyes. I felt anxious when they did this. None of the nurses addressed me after the procedure, and I did not question them about their findings. But something made me feel anxious. Anxious enough not to tempt fate by asking if Neil's body was responding in all the right ways. But I think I had an intuition that something might be wrong.

After a time, a young male nurse who had so far not been assigned to Neil became one of our regular nurses. I liked him immediately. He was professional, polite, friendly and obviously very bright. I heard from one of the older nurses in the CCU that he planned to enter medical school in the fall. I watched him perform the usual routine one afternoon, and while he was sweeping the light across Neil's eyes he murmured, without looking at me, "He doesn't seem to be able to see..."

I received the blow like a life sentence I did and didn't expect. The only sound I heard was the roar of complete silence—an isolating silence that whooshes you out of the here-and-now and envelopes you in all-encompassing static generated from your own ears. What could I say? In what manner could I possibly respond to his observation? Was he throwing out a question or announcing a new, cruel, unfathomable, life-altering fact?

While I can see the entire tableau in detail—the young male nurse with flashlight in hand, Neil, comatose in a white hospital bed, the stone statue that is me, Alison —I have no memory of what happened directly afterward. A clicking collage of vignettes has taken the place of a linear sequence of events. Time became wavy and warped with some pieces elaborately stretched out and others shrunk to non-existent.

In one image I arrive in Neil's darkened room early in the morning. On his lap is the white board. I gaze down at his wispy attempt to communicate. Some of the letters are piled on top of their neighbors, but I can decipher seven heart-breaking words: "I cant see I am so sad." Next, I am out in front of our motel with Jim, the endless snow falling, and I say in a mad-at-the-universe voice, "I can't BELIEVE that Neil is blind!" and Jim says nothing to refute me or to indicate that I am over-reacting like I hoped he would. In another, I am standing in a corner with one of the interns from Neurology, and he says,

"There is nothing on Neil's MRI that indicates that he is blind." And Dr. Renaud walks in and offers that it is possible that this situation is temporary, and I say, "Well that's what I'm counting on." And then I see myself, tears streaming down my face, Jim beside me by Neil's bed and Dr. Carrington on the other side. He decides to insert a monitor into Neil's forehead to assess whether or not there is inter-cranial pressure that may be causing the problem. In one snapshot I am talking on the phone to my sister, Lesley, telling her everything. And she says to me, "If it turns out that Neil is blind, he will learn to live his life in a different way. And it will be a good life." I ask, "Do you really think that's true?" And she says, "Absolutely." In the next slide, I round a corner and there is my Judy walking toward me, out of nowhere. She says, "I know I didn't call, but Jessica told me to get in the car and just drive up." She, Jim and I eat lunch in the hospital cafeteria, and during the entire meal I sit there, amid all the other diners, openly weeping and weeping with no regard for the setting. And they reiterate Lesley's words, while making no attempt to get me to pull myself together. And in the final scene, I am beside myself, not unlike the afternoon of our first conference with Dr. Renaud in the little room off the CCU waiting room. I turn to Jim in my anguish and I cry, "How much more can we take?" And he looks me straight in the eye and answers, "As much as they dish out."

∼

In the midst of our shock and grief, Neil began to show some evidence of physical progress. The respiratory specialist stopped in one day as I sat by Neil's bedside. He pointed to the monitor at the head of the bed and told me that it indicated that Neil was doing most of his breathing on his own. The machine was doing very little to support him now, and the time had come to once again remove the breathing tube and watch how he handled it. So the test date was scheduled, and Neil failed again, sputtering and choking as he had before. He simply had not healed to the point where his body could function on automatic. His breathing was completely compromised without some type of support. Dr. Carrington decided that the time had come to order a tracheotomy. If Neil's breathing could not take place above his neck like it was supposed to, then it would have to temporarily take place below it until his body relearned what we all take for granted. The next day, Neil was fitted with a brand new tube which sprouted from his throat. It was, indeed, his ticket out of the CCU and back up to Neurology from where he'd started, weeks ago.

Upon his arrival in the Neurology wing, Neil was fitted with another apparatus: a stomach tube. Now all his nutrients, in the form of Ensure, could be poured directly into this tube several times a day. He was a new man, with tubes protruding from different areas than before. The one in his throat, the trache, allowed him more freedom of movement, something he had not experienced in weeks on the breathing tube, but it was not without its own set of challenges. Neil had to learn how to live with and use the trache. It allowed him to breathe independently, but the pooling of fluid at the entrance to his throat was still a huge issue. His mouth had to be suctioned out, something that the nurses did regularly until he eventually learned how to spit the fluid into a paper towel—one more step toward independence.

∾

March 1, 2008 was my sixtieth birthday. Being a seemingly permanent resident of University-North Medical Center in the midst of a life trauma is never how anyone imagines spending such a milestone. I was really down. On the drive to the hospital the phone rang. It was a friend, letting me know that she was thinking of me on my special day. How could I not express my despair? She said, "I've definitely heard of cases such as Neil's where sight is regained after a period of vision loss. It's entirely possible that Neil will see again." As I hung up, I thought, "Happy Birthday, Alison. You've just been given a gift. It may not be what you wanted, but it will do for now." The gift, of course, was Hope. I held it close to me all day long.

As soon as we arrived at the hospital, Jim headed to Neil's room and I headed in the other direction to get our coffee. As I carried the two steaming cups down the hallway toward Neil's room, Jim intercepted me before I entered. He was clearly excited, almost bursting with an unexpected surprise for me.

"Honey!" he cried, "Neil can talk! He wants to show you something!"

I was totally unprepared for this surprise, this other

March 1st milestone. Although we had never discussed the issue of Neil's verbal communication, with the way our story was unfolding, we both had come to believe that additional blows were a distinct possibility. Perhaps Neil had been robbed of the ability to speak along with the loss of his vision. I entered the room and said, "Hi Neil."

I watched Neil put his hand to his throat and plug the hole of his tracheotomy with his finger. In a raspy, kind of slurred voice he said, "Happy Birthday, Mom."

I leaned down and put my arms around his now narrow shoulders and held him close to my heart. He hugged me back, blocked the air flow from the trache again and said, "You look even younger this year than you did last year."

I laughed and tightened my hold on my gift. Happy Birthday to me.

*n*MY COMMUNICATION SKILLS HAD CONSISTED of nodding or shaking my head and labored attempts at writing on a whiteboard. My next leap in communication was made possible by that inanimate little object, the trache tube, inserted into my neck just below my throat. I was deemed ready for the trache after my body got the hang of breathing without outside help and, for me, it was a savior, providing one of the only times I felt a glimmer of hope during my long stay at University-North.

When most people think of undergoing a tracheotomy, they probably grimace and shield their vulnerable throats in a protective manner. Maybe they envision an older guy who contracted throat cancer due to a three pack a day habit who now must block his trache hole in order to speak, and they hope that that fate will never be theirs. While I may have shared this response earlier in my life, I now look back on the trache as a sort of holy grail that I took a perilous quest to find, even though it was simply installed by a doctor. The gift this little tube bestowed on me was the ability to speak at last, and Hallelujah for that! I was grateful beyond measure to have the air tube days behind me. I should probably qualify my statement to say that the trache allowed me to practice speaking, the imperative word being "practice," as half my face was, and still is, completely paralyzed. This situation made it hard to have the proper control over my lips and tongue—to make them coordinate and go in the right direction. But I had been silenced for so long that it was satisfying enough to hear myself talking even if everyone else had to concentrate hard to understand what the hell I was saying.

When I was awake and alert I was anxious to communicate with anyone who was willing to decipher what I was trying to say, whether it was a loved one or a hospital employee sent in to empty the contents of my catheter tube. It didn't matter. I just needed to connect. And when there was no one else around and I had the energy, I would talk out loud to myself.

Despite the progress that the trache afforded me, I couldn't stand that half my mouth was paralyzed, causing me to drool constantly. In my mind there is some sort of parallel between drooling and dopiness. It conjures the image of my uncle's golden retrievers, two somewhat vapid creatures. They are mindlessly happy with huge ropes of drool hanging from their mouths. I certainly did not want to resemble them, but I found it impossible to swallow my own saliva. Most people never know, never ponder, the ridiculous issue of how much spit we create. Everyone just unconsciously swallows and it's gone—nothing to it. But without the ability to handle this task, the saliva accumulates at the back of the throat, and there is no other option than to manually clear it out. But, hey —one giant leap forward, one baby step back.

NEIL STAYED IN THE NEUROLOGY UNIT for ten days. Although his body still needed healing sleep throughout the day, he definitely was awake more and more. It was time to investigate his vision loss, and he was scheduled to be examined in Ophthalmology. He had two appointments during this period. Jim was present for one of them, and for one he was escorted by the beautiful young nurse.

When I arrived in Neurology on the morning that she transported him, they were not yet back from the appointment. I waited for them in the small room with the large window overlooking the hall where weeks before I had watched her push him on the gurney to the operating room. I didn't have long to wait before I saw them emerge from the elevator. They were not communicating. There was no camaraderie or chit chat. Each faced straight ahead in complete silence. I knew immediately that things had not gone well. I watched her wheel him into his room and emerge. I approached her as she headed to the nurses' station where she confirmed what I already knew. The appointment had not gone well. The news was bad, and Neil appeared to be withdrawn and depressed. She said, "You should go in. He probably needs you."

I entered his room and said, "Neil, I hear that the appointment didn't go well. I'm so, so sorry."

I gathered him in my arms and laid my head on his. I kissed the long pink scar which stretched from the top of his head to the front of his ear. My heart ached for this child of mine. I had given him life and for what? To have it so cruelly altered from one of promise and bright horizons to one of bitter disappointment and endless darkness? I didn't think I could stand it. But I knew I had to for Neil. I had to pretend to be strong and calm. I had to transmit this state to him. From the recesses of my broken heart, my barely functional mind, I could see my role, my job, beginning to take shape. My mission was coming into focus, revealing itself to me.

"Neil, I would give my life for you." I could feel the tears come, making my eyes blink and burn.

"I know," he whispered. "It's OK."

He let go of me and lay back on his pillow. He laced his hands together over his chest and shut his eyes. In less than a minute he had fallen asleep—the only escape available to him.

n THERE WAS NO WAY I COULD believe my blindness was permanent. I mean, come on —this nightmare had to be a side effect of trauma from the surgery—temporary trauma. I had to cling to this possibility and the conviction that it would right itself with a little time. I just had to be patient and I would heal, regain my vision. But, as days and weeks passed, I began to feel more anxious. I wasn't getting any better. At times, I could swear that I'd just seen something; for a fleeting second or two I could see again—my vision had returned, just like I'd heard that it could. I wanted to see so badly that, in retrospect, I believe my mind was playing tricks on me.

*a*JIM TOLD ME THAT DR. SHERIDAN, the ophthalmologist who examined Neil over two visits, had wished she could do something that would "fix" Neil. If an operation existed that would remedy his vision loss, she would have him in an operating room in a heartbeat. However, it appeared that the life had literally been squeezed out of his optic nerves. Rather than looking rich and red, the result of being fed by nourishing blood, they were completely pale and lifeless. This diagnosis was later confirmed at Massachusetts Eye and Ear, where Mia took Neil for a second opinion.

The die was cast there and then in those last ten days at University-North, although neither Neil nor I could fully integrate this knowledge. We understood what had been explained to us, but we were not capable of really and truly believing it. We had allowed hope to enter our psyches, to seep into our cells, and I don't think that it's possible for it to simply drain out like the sucking swoosh of water down the drain once the plug has been pulled. Some droplets of hope get left behind. They linger.

They only dry up gradually the way rain evaporates eventually from a full, shimmering puddle. It takes time.

Neil saw Dr. Sheridan once a year for the first few years of his blindness; he no longer does. A few years ago, he asked her if she thought that somehow, somewhere down the line, medical advances, including stem cell research, might make it possible to regenerate an optic nerve, thereby restoring at least some of his sight. Her response was that research is happening all the time in this vast new field, and some day it probably will be possible.

We know, of course, that "some day" is not definable. But just in case it should ever appear on the horizon, Neil is taking very good care of his eyes. He makes sure they are protected from the sun and adequately lubricated. We don't waste our days ever discussing it. The puddle of hope within us is pretty well evaporated by now. But a droplet or two may still exist in some shady recess.

I WAS IN A MISERABLE STATE during my endless days at University-North Medical Center. I couldn't think about my life. I was too scared to do it. All I saw was darkness, both literally and symbolically. I felt like I was trapped in a dark theater as the performance ends. The curtain is pulled tight, the lights dim out to total blackness. The show is over. But, for some reason, I cannot get up and find the Exit. I can't walk into the light just outside the theater.

I couldn't help but dwell on the life I left behind. And

leaving it behind was exactly what had happened. I had had no choice but to jump in the car and speed up north to this hospital, leaving everything in my wake—no tearful good-byes, no closure of any sort. I was just gone. A few times I'd awake with a start, in a nightmarish state in my hospital bed, thinking I was back at Greenwood School, paranoid that I had overslept. I'd missed "wake up" and the kids were still in bed, my surrogate sons. They were supposed to be in first period class by now. I felt frantic. Then reality would sink in, and I was engulfed in sadness. I felt such a huge loss, as though someone or something evil had broken into the dorm and kidnapped my boys from under my nose. But the sad fact was that I had abandoned them, though unwillingly. All I wanted was to go back, to be surrounded by the boys I had come to love and who loved me back. How were they holding up without me?

There was no way of imagining any kind of future for myself. Where was my life supposed to go from here? What was I supposed to do?

*a*NOW IN NEUROLOGY, WITH A LITTLE more freedom of movement possible, the physical therapists began to rotate Neil's rag-like body to a sitting position on the edge of his bed with his feet touching the floor, an event that had not occurred in what seemed a lifetime. In order to do this, one of them pulled his body up while the other climbed onto the bed behind him to push and swivel him. This "uprightness" was the obvious next step on their list of goals. During the first couple of sessions, the minute the PTs took their hands off him, Neil would simply flop over. His strength, balance, and muscle tone had seriously atrophied.

His weakness in this department, however, was counterbalanced by his total commitment to work at whatever challenge was put to him and his determination to succeed. He was every physical therapist's dream patient—weak in body and strong in willpower. Before long they hoisted him to his feet using a wide cotton belt, put him behind a walker, and practiced walking down the hallway toward the nurses' station. My job was to follow behind carrying a chair. In case Neil's strength gave out, I could quickly plunk down the chair to offer him a rest. It was great insurance, but he never needed it. With the nurses cheering him on, Neil soon worked up to doing multiple laps around their station, accompanied by a PT or a strong male nurse. He had also reached the point of sitting in a chair for part of each day rather than being confined to his bed.

After so many weeks of unconsciousness and serious setbacks, Neil was inching his way forward, despite his traumatic loss of vision. Nevertheless, I was completely taken by surprise when a hospital planner approached me to say that it was time for Neil to move on from University-North, and we needed to make some decisions regarding the next step. What in the world was she talking about? He was weak, blind, took nourishment through a stomach tube, and relied on a tracheotomy to breathe? Was she out of her mind?

She explained to me that a hospital setting was no longer

the place for Neil. He was physically stable and needed to move to a rehabilitation facility where he would receive many more hours of the kind of work he was doing with the hospital physical therapists. That is what rehab centers do. His leaving the hospital with both stomach and trache tubes were issues that rehab settings were equipped to handle. She had already made contact with the southern office of Vermont Division for the Blind and Visually Impaired, and the director was prepared to meet Neil once he had settled into his next facility.

I was completely unsettled. It was not that I didn't understand what she was saying to me. And it was not that what she explained didn't make sense. I just had never thought much about the separate, specialized work of medical hospitals versus rehabilitation hospitals. I never expected in this whole arduous journey to include a step called "rehab." I had wrapped my mind around serious surgery for a large, malignant brain tumor, then treatment for the remaining cancer. All this was staggering enough. It sucked the breath from my body when I allowed it to really sink in. But I simply was unprepared for being dismissed, shoved out, in such a sad and broken state.

My son had entered this hospital with a ticking time bomb embedded in his skull, it's true. But he had entered walking, talking, breathing, and seeing—a seemingly normal twenty-eight year old who needed immediate surgery and follow-up treatment for brain cancer. As grim as that scenario was, I could never, even in my overactive, worrier's imagination, have envisioned his current state. And now, in my own fragile state, the hospital seemed to be saying, "This is what you get. This is the best we could do. It's someone else's turn." It just felt so damn final. Our lives had been ransacked—were completely unfamiliar to us—and we had no idea how to reclaim them.

Somehow, however, albeit in a blur, we managed to regroup, to put one foot in front of the other, and with grit and resolve prepared to move on to the next phase of this supreme test. Neil's life was on the line, and together we had to pick up the pieces, rearrange them as best we could, with positive energy, hope, and trust that we would find our way.

*n*THE ONLY THING GOING FOR ME as far as my mental health was concerned—the reason I didn't go positively crazy — was that everything, in my perception at least, was happening so fast I didn't have time for processing: news of the tumor, being overtaken by seizures, my dependence on an oxygen tube lodged in my throat, being unable to communicate or to see. It all came on in such breakneck speed. I know the days dragged on in slow motion for my family, but for me, time was different. When you find yourself dealing so suddenly with a life-threatening, life-altering condition, everything spins out of control, causing you to lose your balance. In a blink you find yourself in a hospital bed, being pushed down long, strange hallways, and you cannot fully grasp what is happening. It just doesn't make sense. You are simply not in a place to think about anything on the grand scheme of things. By the time you can process each piece of awful news, it has become a reality you are forced to adjust to. You have to pull yourself together with your wits in working order.

I suppose an additional reason for my not falling too far into a bottomless pit of despair was that there was constant energy surrounding me. It is hard to linger in introspection when you are always being interrupted. Between the cheerful nurses showing up on a regular schedule to take vitals, loved ones coming to surround me with their healing spirits, physical therapists working to loosen my rusted-up body, I didn't have much time during the day to sink into despair. But, you might ask, what about the long nights of lying alone in the never-ending darkness? How is it possible to battle despair when questions such as "What if you discovered the tumor earlier?" or "What will you do if you never regain your sight?" push you into the dreaded dark places.

Believe me, my mind could and did migrate to to those places. But, to be honest, during that time I was too damned tired to think about much of anything at all. Sleep was my solace, my escape, and my necessity. I had no idea before those hospital days that fatigue had levels beyond which I'd experienced. The fatigue I felt after all I'd endured was totally different from being simply tired or burnt out or even exhausted. It was truly like being "lifeless." Right in front of me the most engaging spectacle could be unfolding—the Superbowl, a strip show, my twin brother's newborn baby—it wouldn't have mattered. When this overwhelming fatigue seeped into every cell in my body, I was not available to watch, to participate, to even lift an eyelid.

∽

While it didn't make me happy—nothing at this point could have made me happy—I learned some news that encouraged me to focus on my rehabilitation. I was finally being released from University-North Medical Center, my place of residence for the last six weeks. It came as a relief to me and I think also for my parents who had chosen to stay by my side far from home. Now they'd be able to sleep in their own bed and see me every day at my new temporary home, the rehabilitation wing at Southside Medical Center in southern New Hampshire.

The best thing about the news was that it meant that I was making progress: I had gained the ability to breathe on my own with the assistance of a trache tube; I could sit up for longer periods of time and even walk with the aid of a walker. These were the accomplishments that allowed me to move closer to home to a more local hospital without quite the massive presence of University-North.

ON MARCH TENTH, THE DAY BEFORE Neil's twenty-ninth birthday, he and Mia were transported by ambulance to southern New Hampshire, thirty-five minutes from our home. Jim and I followed behind in the car. As we drove south, I remember thinking that we had made it through the darkest of days—dark for Jim and me, Jessica, Jackson, and Mia. But the dark days for Neil stretched endlessly ahead.

FIVE

MOVING ON

Sadness

You mustn't be frightened
if a sadness
rises in front of you.
Larger than any you have ever seen;
if an anxiety, like light and cloud-shadows
moves over your hands
and over everything you do.
You must realize that something
is happening to you,
that life has not forgotten you,
that it holds you in its hand
and will not let you fall.

~ Rainer Maria Rilke

AS THE DAY APPROACHED, I BEGAN feeling both ready and glad to leave University-North and everything that it stood for in my life—all that it had cost me, even though I knew, full well, that it had also saved my life. What I wanted to do, however, was to shake it off like a dog shakes off a greedy flea which sucks some of its life blood. I wanted to shake myself clean and leave its enormity behind. While I realized that University-North would continue to be a formidable presence in my new life—probably always would be—it felt good to be checking out as a long-term resident. The fact that I was exchanging a hospital bed there for another one a little closer to home in a rehab hospital felt like a step in the right direction, even if it was no more than a baby step.

*a*I WILLED MYSELF TO THINK THAT Neil's move to the rehabilitation wing at Southside Medical Center was a positive move in the right direction. It took enormous willpower to muster any happiness about anything that was occurring in our lives. I couldn't give thanks that Neil was out of danger—that journey had not even begun. I couldn't breathe a sigh of relief that Neil was close to getting his former life back. That would probably never happen. If I had to articulate a goal at all it might have been to build up Neil's strength and endurance in order to begin a year of treatment to overcome the remaining malignancy in his brain. But that goal was at the lower end of the priority list as we pulled into the Southside parking lot. The goal at hand, as I saw it, involved a different type of survival altogether, and it was this: to do whatever it took to keep Neil from giving up on his life; to figure out how to forge something new that would be worth living; to surround him with tender yet fierce love that sends the message—we believe in you, your strength, your resilience, your courage. You are our son and we will be by your side for whatever mountain you are required to climb. You will never be alone. Now start climbing.

We had been told that all the rooms at Southside were

double occupancy. Neil would have a roommate, something we were not used to during the endless weeks at University-North when we formed permanent family encampments in Neil's spacious, light-filled rooms. Somehow, we would adjust to our new situation, our new surroundings. We were flexible.

By the time Jim and I arrived at Southside, Neil had been admitted. We found him propped up in his new bed and Mia unpacking his personal belongings. We exchanged pleasantries with the elderly man in the adjacent bed who was watching TV, and in short order several nurses arrived, pulled the privacy curtain, and proceeded to socialize with us in an effort to get to know Neil, assess his situation, and fill him in on the services and schedule that would make up this next stage of his life.

The nurses on duty that night were great—lively and positive and welcoming. They told Neil he'd be seeing a physical therapist, a speech and language therapist, an occupational therapist, even a "recreational" therapist. He would meet these practitioners the next day, his birthday.

The move had gone smoothly. As Jim and I prepared to leave for the night, I felt gratitude—gratitude that Neil was in good hands, that he had made it to the next step, that I would get up in the morning and have a shorter drive to this new facility, that Neil had work in front of him that would take time and effort and commitment, work that he was equal to and eager to start. I understood, at least in that moment, that the way I had to live was "one step at a time." And somehow I had to help my formerly fast-moving, twenty-nine year old son see that living this unfamiliar way was entirely possible.

*n*THE RIDE DOWN TO SOUTHERN New Hampshire was a journey of non-stop discomfort. I was strapped to a backboard and buckled into an ambulance. Almost immediately I felt as though I'd been fastened over a slab of granite, and I remember thinking, "Why is this necessary? I'm not the guy I was six weeks ago, but I don't have a back or neck injury!"

It didn't take long to figure out why being restrained was in my best interest. It was the end of winter, and each highway and byway we traveled was buckled by frost heaves notorious to New England. Like always, they'd flatten out in the coming months, but now they were still rough enough to have dangerously tipped me from side to side had I not been strapped down. But despite the benefit of my restraints, I felt as though I was a can of soda, one that was being endlessly shaken, and by the time we arrived at Southside Medical Center I was ready to explode.

But here I was—finally released to a new facility waiting to rehabilitate all the parts of me that could possibly be rehabilitated. Which was exactly what I was on board to do. I needed to get out of bed and onto my own two feet. That didn't seem like such a tall order, even with my justifiable depression due to my loss of sight and deep frustration with the left side of my body which still exhibited significant weakness.

Despite my sorry state, I was never willing to give up on the idea of rehabilitation. There was not going to be some huge emotional dilemma where they couldn't get me out of bed because

I'd wrapped myself in a fetal position endlessly crying and sucking on my damn thumb. No, not me. I was stronger than that. I knew that if I tried hard enough, I could heal myself. I had to totally believe in and devote myself to the process of healing. That was my grand plan.

a WHEN I ARRIVED THE NEXT MORNING at Southside, I was told that Neil was moving rooms. "Why?" I wondered. Did they not think that Neil was a good fit with his elderly roommate? Were we troublesome or bothersome in some way? I was surprised, seeing how we had only arrived the night before. How much damage could we have done? The nurses, however, were just as cheerful and pleasant as they had been the night before. If they were thinking "problem," it certainly did not show. They did tell me that the beautiful young nurse from University-North had spoken to them to give them the necessary transfer information. She had also relayed that Neil's family was very involved and ever-present. Who knows, she might have mentioned that we take up a lot of space. In any event, there were empty rooms on the floor. The Southside staff thought that Neil would do better in a room of his own, and so, as luck and probably networking would have it, we found ourselves in another large, spacious room with two beds and a lovely woodsy view. We had a new home away from home.

I have powerful memories from our days in southern New Hampshire. One or two make me smile. And many evoke an indescribable sadness. Coming to terms with what is "real" while gripping the lifeline of hope is a formidable challenge. It is confusing and disorienting to slip in and out of each mind state. "Why don't I get it," I remember thinking. "How is it that I get whacked and smacked and the scab on my heart gets freshly pulled off again and again making healing completely impossible?"

Such a moment occurred the second morning I strode into Neil's new room. After hugging him hello, my eyes rose to the white board above his head where the nurses wrote instructions and messages to each other as they changed shifts. Written in large red print was this: "Neil is blind. Make sure you connect verbally—explain procedures, etc."

The sign was too real for me to handle. "No!" I wanted to scream. "If you write that down for the world to see, it must mean that you believe he really is blind—that this life sentence is permanent, forever." I wanted to run from the room screaming. I wanted to be transported to a kinder reality, to an alternate plane of existence. But because moving on with our life was my goal, my resolution, my mission, I swallowed my scream and calmly asked Neil, "How about going out for a walk?"

And Neil had his own tough moments, I know. One morning I'd gotten off to a late start. I walked into his room at ten o'clock, and he had already been up for a long time, had showered, been fed, and was waiting, always waiting. He was sitting in a chair with his head down. The despair in his voice broke my heart anew—yanked the scab again: "I can hear everyone out in the hall, talking and laughing, and I'm alone in here in the dark."

"Well, you're not alone anymore," I replied, "because here I am." And once again we would corral our misery and work at shifting our moods. Sometimes it took supreme effort on both of our parts. But acting the way we wished we felt had definite power, and usually, before long, we were the ones talking and even laughing.

~

The best times at Southside were when Neil was busy working with his rehab team. He was determined to regain his physical strength and balance and to work on his weak left side, which included the left side of his mouth and his left hand. In addition to these goals, it was good for him to be engaged with others. Any work toward rehabilitation, any social contact with his therapists uplifted his spirits. Witnessing Neil's resolve created a little space in my own psyche. The ever-present heaviness in my heart was lightened a bit by the energy of his purpose. Neil was still Neil. His personality, his social giftedness, his appreciation for all that he was receiving brought out great energy and commitment in the professionals who worked with him. They all loved him.

Neil and I had always been into words. We were the only ones in our family who truly loved Scrabble and the word scrambles in the daily newspaper. Our favorite games were dictionary games like Balderdash in which you had to write convincing but incorrect definitions to little known words in an effort to fool everyone else playing. In short, we both loved anything to do with language. So it was not surprising that Brenda, the speech and language pathologist, became a favorite, and both of us looked forward to the times she was scheduled to work with Neil.

The "language" part of Brenda's job was to assess what damage had been done to Neil's memory and to his ability to understand and process language following his brain surgery. I think it was a given that it was unlikely for anyone to emerge from this operation completely unscathed. In our daily interactions I could not really see any obvious holes in Neil's abilities. I was relieved to observe that he seemed cognitively intact. However, once Brenda began her work, I did notice that there were indeed some areas of weakness.

One of the exercises they engaged in was story retelling. Brenda would read a story to Neil, and his job was to answer the questions she asked him following the reading. I noted that many of the stories were pretty low quality—both convoluted and boring at the same time. They actually had the effect of making my mind wander, and I remember feeling fortunate that I was not the one being tested. Nevertheless, I did see, for the first time, that Neil was exhibiting some memory problems. I was surprised that I hadn't been aware of this on my own, felt concerned about it, and at the same time was glad that this issue was being addressed by a highly qualified and dedicated professional. Neil totally enjoyed the sessions. He never felt frustrated as Brenda was so supportive, so optimistic. He loved the challenge, the attention, and the fact that the more time they spent on this work, the sharper he got. Brenda told me that Neil began their sessions at about 70% intact and by the time he left Southside had improved to nearly 100%.

Neil's favorite language activity with Brenda was, naturally, the word games. She would give him a word like "block," and he would have to come up with as many different meanings for the word as he could and use each meaning in an appropriate sentence: "The child put the last block on the tower; the player was able to block the pass; I'll walk down the block to meet you; my possessions will be put on the block at the auction next week." Because Neil was so eager, so engaged, so quick, Brenda had as much fun as he did. She had a lovely, open manner and often included me in the exercises. For both Neil and me, her sessions were a respite from our gloom. They were rays of sunlight penetrating the dark clouds. And we gratefully lifted our faces and basked in the warmth.

*n*AFTER MY FIRST SESSION OR TWO with Brenda it was obvious I had suffered some brain damage following my surgery. My short term memory was shaky at best. I had a hard time holding onto simple memories. Mom would come in in the morning and ask what I'd done the evening before, who had stopped by to visit, and I couldn't immediately remember. I found that I really had to concentrate to retrieve this information; it would take me some time. Then all of a sudden it would come to me, accompanied by a deep sadness for my obvious deficit.

Brenda and I worked on all sorts of memory exercises in order to reawaken and strengthen the part of my brain that stores short term memories. She would read me a paragraph, and I would recount it as accurately and with as much detail as I could. Or she would read me a longer story and ask specific questions related to it: What was the name of the farmer's dog? What kinds of vegetables were grown on the farm? In the end, why did the farmer feel he had to sell the farm?

I had some gaps and joked that if Southside held a remedial memory class for the old timers and the surgical brain patients, I'd be in the front row. Luckily, I showed improvement almost immediately, and Brenda's accolades helped to raise my inner bar. It was such a relief to be successful. I could barely remember what it felt like.

The word games we played actually revealed how intact my brain was in some specific areas. I aced the "multiple uses of a single word" game from the get-go, maybe because I always loved words and word games. Mom and I continued to play and test each other for the sheer fun of it long after I left the rehab center. Try it yourself with the word "run" and see if you can come close to the almost thirty different uses in the dictionary!

AS A SPEECH AND LANGUAGE THERAPIST, Brenda also worked with Neil on the physical side of his speech. The left side of Neil's face had been left paralyzed after the surgical removal of the majority of his tumor. His forehead didn't wrinkle on that side, his eye didn't shut properly on that side, and his mouth was unable to change position on that side. This last inability made for slurred speech, especially when Neil was tired. Not only is slurred speech difficult to understand, it also leaves an unfavorable impression on a listener who may not realize the reason for the slurring. This situation was essential to address and rehabilitate to the fullest degree possible. Brenda had many simple tools and exercises to help Neil, from having him press the inside of his slack cheek with a spoon to make him become aware of that area, to manipulating a button on a string from one side of his mouth to the other and back.

Whatever exercise Brenda taught, Neil diligently practiced during the times between sessions. It was extremely important to him. It is gratifying to note that over time—many months, in fact—Neil's speech improved greatly until his clarity returned to almost normal. After leaving Southside and its regimen of rehab sessions, Neil continued to practice the exercises on his own at home. There were times, especially when he was fatigued, when Jim and I would have to say, "Neil, you're slurring" or "Neil—articulate." He never held it against us, never lashed out or withdrew. He just redoubled his efforts with his focus intact—to heal, to improve, to move forward.

*n*THINKING BACK, BRENDA HAD HER WORK cut out for her the moment I swung into the parking lot of Southside Medical Center and settled into my new digs on her wing. I was the perfect guinea pig-type subject as I had so many issues. I was a speech and language pathologist's dream. Brenda got to practice the full array of her training on me, all at once. Together we addressed the cognitive, the mechanical, and the instinctive/involuntary aspects of my problems—all in three weeks' time.

The mechanical issue was my slurred speech due to the paralysis on the left side of my face. I could talk fine, but I sounded like I'd just downed a six pack of Budweiser. I was ready to address it. I had spent years lifting weights, was used to working my muscles, focusing on and manipulating isolated muscle groups. I'd just never had to do it with my mouth and face. But I was eager to regain what I had lost, so whatever exercises were on Brenda's rehab platter, bring them on!

The button on a string was the mother lode of workouts for a guy with weakness in the jaw, lip, tongue, and inner mouth muscles. The button is the rehab tool, and the string acts, in at least some of the exercises, as a safety precaution—a lifeline to hold onto to keep from accidentally swallowing or choking on the button. Over and over I practiced holding the button, wedged between my teeth on the left side of my mouth and teasing it over to the right side using my tongue and cheeks. That would count as one repetition. My challenge was to count the number of transfers I could achieve in twenty seconds.

Unfortunately, my desire to regain the needed elasticity and my body's pace to do so did not exactly correlate. My motivation was racing down the track at breakneck speed while my physical improvement meandered along. But the gulf between them didn't keep me from working hard. I could barely complete a single repetition in twenty seconds the first dozen or so times I tried. It took longer than twenty seconds to even get a solid feel for the damn button clenched under my teeth let alone move it with my tongue and cheek muscles. It was both frustrating and exhausting. Because it wasn't automatic for me, I tried to use my mind to help isolate the spot on my face, on my lips, that might control these muscles. I wanted to wow Brenda with my progress, my work ethic. I wanted an A for outstanding effort!

Moving on to the next exercise, I'd place the button behind my closed lips, in front of my front teeth. And then I'd slowly but firmly pull on the string, using whatever lip strength I could muster to hold the button in. But the left side of my mouth felt droopy and, sure enough, when I pulled on the string the button would pop out, always from the left. That side was like a lifeless piece of clay. It was like an arm or leg gone numb during the night after sleeping in a strange position. Having cut off the blood circulation temporarily, you wake up to an alien appendage, heavy and lifeless. But unlike a "dead" arm or leg, my problem wasn't temporary. My face would never be symmetrical again. I couldn't see the change in myself, so daily mourning of the loss of my handsomeness didn't weigh on me. There was nothing I could do about that but make up for it with my stellar personality. But I sure as hell wanted to sound like a normal cool guy. So I soldiered on with my button practice.

*a*PERHAPS THE MOST CHALLENGING PART of Neil's work with Brenda was waking up the frozen muscles of his throat and esophagus. He arrived at Southside sporting both his tubes—the trache and the belly tube. He had failed the swallow test more than once before leaving University-North. His body had yet to relearn that automatic reflex and didn't seem to remember that it used to know how! And unlike story recalling or articulation, it was harder to note progress day to day. It seemed more black and white—you could either swallow food or you couldn't. And, so far, Neil couldn't.

Brenda worked with Neil to wake up this natural instinct that had been damaged through surgical trauma. It was hard for me, usually reclined on the bed adjacent to Neil's, to feel much engagement about her instruction and his practice. It wasn't nearly as fun as stories and word games.

*n*THE MOST SUBTLE PART OF MY work with Brenda was the retraining of my throat muscles to swallow—that automatic function that had thrown in the towel for some reason following my surgery. Right away, Brenda started me on an assortment of swallowing exercises in an effort to coax the left side of my throat to begin pulling its weight. I would cover my trache tube with a finger in order to create suction or negative suction—whichever it takes to aid in the process of swallowing. Brenda watched the movements of my Adam's Apple on each attempt, and she would coach me, "Come on, Neil, nope, you can do it—try to focus on those muscles—nope, I'm not seeing it, Neil."

I felt like shouting, "You ain't seeing it cuz I ain't feeling it!" It was obvious to her naked eye that no flexing was happening in the appropriate places. My throat would not do what it had done unconsciously for twenty-nine years, even as I willed it to with everything I had. I'd end each session frustrated. But if Brenda was, she never showed it. She assured me that it would happen, that my body would begin to respond, as it was doing in all the other areas we were working on.

~

I arrived at the rehabilitation wing of Southside Medical Center sporting both a trache tube and a belly tube. However, before leaving University-North I'd mastered the skill of dealing with the saliva that pooled continuously at the back of my throat. I had graduated from needing the nurses to suction me out to spitting the puddle into a tissue or paper towel. I probably used more paper towels than a family of five uses in a year; a small child could drown in the amount of saliva I created in a single day.   It's no wonder to me now that our bodies are ninety percent water!

Through sheer devotion to me, my mom and dad, my siblings and my girlfriend swooped up mountains of paper towel wads in and around my hospital bed and supplied me with fresh ones. They even seemed cheerful, as this distasteful task signified progress on my part. I get a lump in my throat as I pay tribute to their generosity and support by caddying around my gargantuan spitballs and only picking on me a little, proclaiming, "You sure do drool a lot for someone who can't even eat!"

The belly tube was a necessary piece of equipment, allowing me to take nourishment by bypassing the paralyzed parts of me. The gadget was pretty basic, consisting of a clear plastic tube inserted through my abdomen and into my stomach—a direct conduit for liquid food. All that was required of the nurses or my father or Mia was to pour a couple cans of the liquid nutrient into a funnel, watch it disappear down my new appendage, cap me off and I'd be good to go. After mealtime I'd usually say something like, "I found that particular can of Ensure to be full-bodied, yet unassuming," and we'd all get a good laugh. I felt good that I still had the ability to make my family laugh. It's therapeutic to laugh at your life, even if it lies in ruins at your feet.

The belly tube was part of my body for many weeks. And I never had a hunger pang. But I was denied the pleasure of eating real food, of having choices, of using my mouth, my teeth, my throat, my taste buds. I got gypped on the whole food program during rehab. Each morning I'd sit in my room, freshly showered and dressed, listening to the kitchen staff pass by delivering breakfast to other patients. Alongside my sadness that I was suspended in darkness—couldn't people-watch to add an element of interest to the day that lay ahead—was the insult of smelling the tantalizing whiff of fresh coffee and blueberry muffins, sending my olfactory nerves on a roller coaster ride. But all I had on my menu was Ensure and without the benefit of even tasting it. I missed the flavor of food. It's kind of sick to think that during the time I was unable to swallow I was being deprived of yet another sense—the sense of taste. It struck me that I going about five for seven in the area of sense pathways.

~

I would be lying if I didn't admit that Brenda's optimism and unflagging encouragement were major highlights in my life. She had a way of making me feel like her star student, and maintaining her high opinion of me became a primary goal. I could not yet fully grasp, let alone handle, the way my life was unfolding and the challenges that faced me down the line. So I took on what I could—short term goals like pleasing my teacher and putting my all into tasks I had a chance of accomplishing.

And Brenda was right, all along. Slowly, so slowly that at first I didn't notice, my throat began dealing with much of the saliva that I had been spitting into tissues. If I wondered at first if I was right about this, I actually had proof, for the mountains of spit rags that accumulated around my bedside began to shrink in size with each passing day. Everyone noticed it, commented on it, took it as a positive sign, and so did I. It was as if my tight, rigid muscles had relaxed, and the saliva, instead of backing up, was beginning to make its way down my unlocked throat.

Once I noticed this change I began to practice swallowing on my own. I did it privately, when I was alone in my room, as I was so used to failing in front of others who wanted me to feel success and happiness in any small step of my rehabilitation. It would take a couple of minutes and the utmost concentration, but one evening I was convinced I felt a small swallow. As modest as it was, it gave me just enough drive to keep practicing.

During our session the day after this mini breakthrough I told Brenda about my behind-the-scenes success. She was excited but, of course, she wanted to see evidence of it. As she positioned herself in front of my Adams Apple, performance anxiety crept into every crevice of me. I felt like everyone in the entire hospital was watching and holding their collective breath. I pictured old patients emerging momentarily from their comas, new born babies sucking in their first cry, visitors, conversing with their hospitalized loved ones, breaking off mid sentence—all anxiously awaiting my small miracle. I stood in silence before Brenda, asking my throat muscles to demonstrate what I had reported to her. Brenda's concerned voice broke my concentration: "Neil, are you all right?" I held up my hand, assuring her that I just needed a little more time—and then it happened.

Brenda let out a joyous sound in the wake of my Adam's Apple's slow rise and fall, evidence that I had, indeed, swallowed. And even now that I have joined the ranks of those who take this involuntary action for granted, I will never forget how it felt to unlock those rusted muscles in front of an eager, imaginary crowd.

A day or two following this minor miracle I bid farewell to my trusty, trust-worthy trache tube. It had served me well—afforded me independence to move forward in my rehabilitation. But its necessity and usefulness had played out. I was perfectly capable of keeping myself from drowning in or choking on my own saliva. On Brenda's watch and recommendation a doctor arrived in my room to remove it, and the small hole in my throat closed up almost immediately. So—one tube down and one to go.

Although I had demonstrated there and then that my reflexes were waking up, it didn't mean I could actually swallow anything of substance. Brenda and I both knew this, but she felt it was time to undergo the formal swallow test to assess just how much of my reflex had returned. I knew my new ability was still weak and definitely not automatic, but Brenda was the boss, the decision was made, and the test was scheduled for the following day. I had a hard time falling asleep that night. I woke up once or twice during the night, and when I did, I made myself perform a few practice swallows in preparation for the test.

When Brenda arrived in the morning, I was nervous and expressed doubts that I was ready to be tested. I didn't want to let her down. She assured me in her ever-supportive way that not making it all the way through the test was not the end of the world. It would give us information we needed about my progress and where the areas of difficulty still lay.

We made our way to the basement level of the hospital where the radiologist was set up and waiting for us. Brenda led me to a chair and told me that to my right was a screen where she would watch the x-ray images of my mouth and esophagus doing the work we hoped they'd do. And to my left were several small plates of food which would serve as my test samples. She then backed up to view the screen and left me on stage with the technician who served as both waiter and machine operator.

Sample number one was a tiny cup of pudding, considered

the easiest substance to handle. I remember thinking, "Are you kidding? I love pudding—it practically swallows itself. You don't even have to chew the stuff. It simply slides down your throat, sweet and easy." I could feel my nervousness begin to melt.

But there was a hitch. The pudding was "contaminated" in a way that turned my stomach, for each little sequential hors d'oeuvre included in the test was liberally smeared with a pasty substance called barium, hence the name Barium Swallow Test. Barium is a soft, silvery-white alkali earth metal that is magnetic. Its use in the swallow test was to ensure that each food item would be visible via live x-ray so that therapists like Brenda could witness the mechanics of eating. Its properties allow the bolus—a chewed up wad of food—to be tracked on its journey from mouth to stomach. In addition, once the esophagus gets coated with the barium, it can be observed for signs of contraction. And, unfortunately, what Brenda witnessed that morning was that my muscles were still not up to the task before them.

The pudding was much less forgiving than I'd imagined. With barium in the mix it felt like a thick glob of rubber cement. I did my best but realized in pretty short order that there was no way it was going down, so in an act of utter shame I spit it out. How discouraging. I couldn't even swallow the easiest sample. It was obvious I didn't stand a chance with anything in the solid range. My test ended after sample one, and although Brenda had said it wouldn't be the end of the world, to me it was. All the practicing had done me no good. It was true that my brain was now sending the message to the appropriate muscles in my throat.

They just hadn't developed the strength to swallow anything more than my own saliva.

I didn't stay down long, however. I consoled myself with the fact that I'd made an essential first step: I had managed to isolate the muscles needed for swallowing. That is exactly what I had been doing for years as a weight lifter, and I had learned from experience that once a muscle "gets" how to contract through muscle memory, it's just a matter of time and continued practice before that muscle will grow stronger and more resilient. I would use that same knowledge now—commit to tirelessly exercising and strengthening my throat muscles. I had roughly a week to get ready for my next test.

On retest day I had some nervousness, not to mention embarrassment about my previous performance. But I also felt more confident as I'd figured out how to lubricate my throat a little before swallowing. This little technique did the trick with the barium-laced pudding. I did it—I downed the pudding success-fully— Yeah, dog!

I was told that the next sample was a square of bacon. I could feel myself salivate as I envisioned bacon the way my grand-mother cooked it, warm and flexible with just the right amount of delectable fat. I knew I could chew it, and the grease would help lubricate my throat without me having to direct my saliva to the area. But, as we know, what our minds cook up and the sad facts of the matter are often on opposite ends of the spectrum because it was pretty obvious that this square of bacon had been lifted from the cafeteria at least an hour before my test. It was stone cold and beyond crisp; it was downright brittle. And, of course, it was smeared with barium. As I chewed and chewed, the bacon transformed into a mucky, fibrous wad of strands—too much for my fledgling throat muscles to receive and dispose of. This time, barium covered bacon was my downfall.

I didn't handle this defeat well. My state of mind must have been obvious to Brenda because after I had wiped myself clean from this latest failed effort and maybe wiped a couple of vagrant tears from my sightless eyes, I felt her sit down beside me and put her arm around my sagging shoulders. I had to admit I was surprised and touched by the divergence from her usual professionalism. I had Brenda pegged as a little straight-laced, a bit of a Girl Scout, someone who didn't often color outside the lines. But I will never forget the next moment. As she commended me on a valiant effort, she slid a little cup into my hand. It was ice cold and familiar-feeling, and I recognized it almost immediately as a dixie cup of ice cream. I could feel the small, flat wooden spoon tucked underneath. She said, "This is against the rules, but here—I'll sit next to you to make sure you can handle it. And here is a regular spoon."

"Good call," I teased, my misery lifting a little. "Watching me eat my first ice-cream in over two months with a tiny wooden stick would be a comedy of errors we both could do without."

I probably made more mess than your typical toddler as I wolfed down this sinfully delectable gift. I think my taste buds had been on the verge of packing it up and calling it quits altogether. Lack of use was causing their atrophy until suddenly and unexpectedly they were bathed in the smoothest, creamiest, sweetest, barium-free substance imaginable. They were alive! And it was thanks to the wonderful Brenda who stuck by my side, even if it meant crossing the line for a minute so her discouraged student could enjoy a good old fashioned childhood treat.

"We'll keep practicing," she said. "We're making progress. I think Time Number Three will be the magic number." I wanted to say, "I think so too," but I could feel a lump forming in my throat and didn't trust myself to say the words. I did, however, nod in agreement.

So now I have a small confession to make, one I couldn't admit to if Brenda was anywhere near my shoulder as I write this. As I predicted, my muscle memory was growing from my continual swallowing practice, and I felt it stronger every day. In tandem with my physical progress was my confidence. I just knew I was "there."

I understood that from Brenda's professional perspective, safety dictated that I not consume anything solid unless and until the process was supervised and observed by a speech and language therapist, but I ended up doing just that—consuming morsels of food, unsupervised and unobserved by a licensed professional.

Jessica had arrived home for a week's visit shortly after my second swallow test. I told her about my miserable failures but that, in the past few days, I thought I'd turned a corner. I felt stronger every day, more in control of my body. And I was almost positive that I now could chew and swallow just about anything put in front of me. So she and I formed a secret alliance.

As we sat alone in my room she kept a lookout, and if the coast was clear, would slip me a bit of the clementine she was eating. I would pretend to cough and while covering my mouth, would pop the morsel of fruit between my lips. The explosion of juice was like heaven, and the remaining skin would slide easily down my throat. We moved on to small chunks of cheese and nickel sized slices of banana, even a crust of bread or two. I can't say I handled everything like a pro, but there was nothing we tried that gave me too much trouble. I told myself that this was practice on an advanced level, and I was being supervised by the big sister I'd always adored and trusted. My heart swells at the memory of this shared time together. And more than the gratitude I felt for my awakening body was the gratitude for Jessica's love for me, the little brother who always had been, and still was, worth going out on a limb for.

Five days later I passed the complete swallow test. I managed both the bacon and a hunk of dry corn muffin iced with the last barium I hope I ever have to endure. It was, for me, a glorious day, another rung up the ladder of reclaiming my body. And I dedicate my victory to the wonderful Brenda with her healing spirit and her eternal optimism . I will always be in Brenda's corner as she was always in mine. And if she is a bit of a Girl Scout, so what? Consider me a lifetime Brownie!

A VERITABLE CROWD ACCOMPANIED NEIL and Brenda to the basement of Southside the morning of his third swallow test. This challenge had now taken on mythic proportions in our lives. But most of us in the peanut gallery that morning—Jim, Jessica, Mia, and I— were more than a little optimistic given Neil's test runs with his big sister. His confidence had rubbed off on us.

As he took a bite from the last plate and began to chew, we held our collective breath, hoping against hope that this dry-looking piece of muffin would embark on its appropriate journey. We watched the screen intently and witnessed the wad swirl and move south down his esophagus in a peristaltic motion like it was descending stairs, one step at a time, in perfect rhythm. Bingo! It was gone.

Brenda jumped up from her chair, hands in the air, as agile as any high school cheerleader, and she let out a whoop before turning and high-fiving us all. She was ecstatic and her enthusiasm was contagious. I, for one, was totally excited for Brenda as well as for Neil. And I was grateful that we, in Neil's family, had had the luxury of witnessing this success with some preliminary confidence and calmness.

Neil was pronounced ready to cautiously enter the world of three squares a day, though it would, in fact, be some time before he could take in enough food by mouth to meet his nutritional needs. It was a happy morning, a tribute to Brenda's personal and professional skill, Neil's unwavering perseverance, the Taylor teamwork, and the human body's ability to relearn and rebuild.

~

At the same time Neil was stretching his mouth, his throat, and his mind with Brenda, he was stretching his body under the tutelage of his physical therapist, Gail. Gail was just Neil's age, almost his height, and a true shepherd in guiding him through his first steps of feeling at home in his body once again.

Neil had spent his whole life as an athlete. He taught himself to ride a two-wheeler at the age of four and excelled at cross-country running in elementary school, winning just about every race he competed in. He was co-captain of his high school lacrosse team and high scorer. He skied, surfed, skateboarded, played tennis, and did extreme mountain biking with a camera strapped to his head to record the harrowing mountain descents he lived through. He and his friends took photos of each other jumping from high rocky cliffs into bodies of water terrifyingly far below. Physical skill and physical thrills were the joy of his life. While I was proud of his abilities—his grace, his coordination, his fearlessness—I was his mother. I always feared for his safety and sometimes questioned his judgment. Worrywart that am, over the years I envisioned an array of horror stories involving crashes or rip tides or severe head injuries. But I never once envisioned Neil's body wasting away from lack of use, his left side weakened from stroke activity and his balance severely compromised by brain surgery and sudden loss of vision. Neil's body was now completely foreign to him.

On the rehab wing of Southside Medical Center everyone needed and received physical therapy to suit their individual circumstances. I have long believed that our bodies are programmed to respond, to heal, to rebuild, to reintegrate. But we all have a ceiling beyond which we probably will not go. Our ceilings are determined by our age, heredity, prior level of fitness, not to mention the condition that necessitated receiving rehab services. For Neil, given his age and who he had been, the ceiling was very high. He was starting at a very low point. And in between, it became apparent, there was huge potential.

When Gail would stride into the room and announce her arrival, Neil would light up, and they'd begin their friendly banter right away. As Neil sat teetering on the edge of his bed, she'd hoist him to standing, and using the PT belt to support him they'd begin the walk down the hall to the PT room. I could hear them laughing as they went, Neil teasing that the day wouldn't be complete without getting his morning wedgie from her.

Gail started slowly with Neil. Much of their early work focused on balance as Neil didn't have much of it and balance is a prerequisite for, let's see...everything! I remember seeing Neil on a ramp with railings on both sides to ensure that he actually remain on the ramp. Gail was never far from him during the earliest days of exercising. Much of the time she was standing right behind him or was actually physically holding him up. But Neil thrived. He always wanted to do more—one more step, one more rep, five more minutes. He would return to his room ready for a nap and yet invigorated by all he had just done. Neil's stay at Southside amounted to just a little over three weeks, so it is remarkable to me that by the end of his stay he would settle into a machine in the rehab room, determined to extend his time from the day before, and Gail would leave him to do his work while she checked on the progress of other patients. Once again, Neil was a success story and an inspiration to all who bore witness to his resolve and to the progress that issued from it.

*n*I IMMEDIATELY FELL IN LOVE WITH MY physical therapist who was a no-nonsense female with a great sense of humor and endless words of encouragement. OK—maybe I wasn't in love in the traditional sense, but even now I smile when I think of her and remember her cheerful morning greeting: "Hey, Neil, it's Gail. Are you ready to roll?" I looked forward to and loved every moment we spent together.

When we first began the program she laid out for me, I wasn't capable of walking unaided. I didn't have the balance to stand alone for more than a few seconds. We made our way to the workout room with her slowly pushing me in a wheelchair and me scuttling my feet along the floor in a walking type motion. In short order, however, I graduated to walking beside Gail, tightly embraced in a PT belt to hold me upright.

Because my balance was so poor, we began the task of building up my legs using a recumbent bike. Each day I'd recline on my butt with my legs extended straight in front of me and just pedal. This was something I could do, and it felt wonderful! Sitting there, pedaling away on my own, I felt free in a way that I hadn't for so long.

I'd pretty much given up on trying to impress Gail with my formidable strength, since I actually had none, but, nevertheless, every day was an improvement from the day before regarding my stamina. I went from four minutes to twelve minutes on the bike—yeehaw! And nothing could stop me.

I knew my balance was still terrible, but I stooped to begging Gail to let me use the stair-stepper machine. To me, it was a big step up from the recumbent bike. Being allowed to exercise in a standing position was, for some reason, a huge deal to me. Maybe I felt that if I was up there standing tall, despite my being in a rehab hospital, no one would know I was sick. Or maybe my butt was starting to hurt from sitting forever on the recumbent bike. Anyway, she finally gave in, maybe swayed by my charm or my pathetic need to impress.

Never would I have guessed that I could get so much joy from an exercise machine! When I was on the lacrosse team in college, we used to laugh at the ridiculous machines that gathered dust in the corner of the weight room. We used free weights and boasted about how much we could bench press or dead lift. If you wanted to build up your legs, then get into the squat rack for a few sets; forget about that sissy machine. We were pretty ignorant and thought we knew more about proper training than we did. I realize that now.

To run on that stair stepper was pure bliss. I could forget about my miserable situation and just run. It was so invigorating. And, ironically, all it took was semi-paralysis on my left side and my blindness for me to see how valuable these wonderful machines are. I should, of course, mention that while I stair-stepped away, Gail was by my side the whole time. She spotted me like a hawk, and if I showed any sign of losing my balance, which was pretty much all the time at first, she would grab the back of my shorts, giving me a massive wedgie. This was our standard mode of safety. I would stride away on the machine with Gail beside it, grasping the back of my shorts in an upward tilt just to keep me steady. She was a tall woman with impressive strength, especially compared to my diminished build. But, hey—I was the one pushing to use the stand-up machines. I could deal with an aggressive means of spotting. So what if I felt like a doll on a ventriloquist's knee. As ridiculous as Gail and I may have looked, I never felt any shame in what I was doing. It was a far cry from glamorous, but it was problem solving that worked for both of us.

What Gail did so well was make me feel we were a team and each new step we took was our next mission. We bonded tightly, as team members do, and I am forever indebted to her wisdom, her kindness, her sensitivity, and the huge role she played in my long journey back to physical fitness.

My life at Southside was in the hands of women, which was not at all bad considering that they were so amazing. Each day started when Elizabeth, the personal care therapist, entered my room to ask if I wanted to bathe. I always said yes. There is nothing as basic, as familiar, as comforting, as a nice hot shower.

I would stand beneath the shower head with my eyes closed, the hot water streaming down my body. With this luxurious, almost decadent experience, came the realization that this was the only part of my day when my blindness and my partial paralysis meant nothing. I was embraced in warmth, a respite from the outside world which felt cold, foreboding, and unrelentingly dark. I was also glad to start each day by washing myself clean of the hospital bed and the general antiseptic smell that comes with hospital living.

Because my balance was still so poor, the wonderful Elizabeth would help me into and out of the shower. She helped me problem solve and practice basic techniques of hygiene in light of the loss of my vision and the weakness of my left side. These were the basics that most people never give a thought to and perform in the privacy of their own bathrooms. But now I had an audience and a coach. Elizabeth taught me how to do the most ungraceful things with a grace I could feel rather than see. I practiced flipping open the top of a shampoo bottle with one hand and squeezing out an appropriate amount with a measure of control. More important than anything, of course, was purposefully remembering where I put each item after using it. We spent much of our time together learning to orient around the bathroom, locating the toilet, the sink, the shower, and the door with my hands or my cane. Elizabeth was with me at the very beginning of the long, challenging, often frustrating process of learning to explore unfamiliar spaces using my tactile sense. This practice felt somewhat like an art form to me, an unfamiliar and now necessary habit I needed to embrace and refine. And over time I have. But in those novice days I felt that never in a million years would I master it.

At first I was a bit modest about getting naked in front of Elizabeth. In my mind, she was an attractive woman, not so much older than I was. At least that's how I envisioned her from the only clues I had to go by—her patient, upbeat nature and her gentle spirit. But after a few days and a couple of awkward showers, my modesty disappeared. There was simply no point in it. I couldn't see myself so what did I care if others saw me in the buff? I had nothing to hide except maybe my annoying drooling which put a small bump in my super-smooth game. So I ended up feeling perfectly comfortable in front of Ellie, as she allowed me to call her. It was her job, after all, to spot my skinny, naked, uncoordinated body while I enjoyed a morning shower. And she was great at it— cheerful, natural, and matter-of-fact.

BY NOW IT WAS LATE MARCH. The endless days of hard winter were winding down and there was promise of spring in the air. March in northern New England is still cold, can still bring snow, but the light is stronger and buds are beginning to swell on the earliest-blooming bushes. Most days, Neil and I bundled up and went outdoors, me pushing him in a wheelchair through the neighborhoods surrounding the hospital. As we walked I described everything we passed—the shapes and colors of the houses, the grass turning greener each day, the dog barking at us from behind the picket fence. I would pick up a pine cone for him to feel, lay his hands on the bark of a tree, stop so we could listen to the high, excited voices of the children on the elementary school playground.

I ask myself now, all these years later, whether I took

any pleasure in those early spring walks with Neil. I do know that a significant portion of my being during that time was consumed with fear for his future, with grief for what was lost, with desperate hope for a miracle to occur, with great pressure regarding how to live the next stage of our lives—the treatment phase—and with my own psychic trauma that manifested as bewilderment and disbelief. A mother was not supposed to be wheeling her once-independent son on daily walks. She should be getting phone calls once a week with messages like, "The coolest thing happened at work today," or "Let's go to a movie—I'll pick you up," or "I'm going camping this week-end, and by the way, I'm getting married!" These walks were such a sad substitution for all the wonderful possibilities that life might have offered. And yet a bond was forged between us that was stronger than anything either of us could ever have imagined. Our walks, our talks, our determination to appreciate the small things we encountered along the way stand out as a gift not everyone gets in a lifetime.

Years ago I read the enthralling and beloved *Little House on the Prairie* series by Laura Ingalls Wilder. While the Ingalls family was living in a particularly unsettled area of Indian territory, they all fell ill with typhoid fever. Every member of the family was in a state of delirium, and the few neighbors who lived near them had to come to their cabin daily to tend to them. While the family recovered, the oldest sister, Mary, awoke to total blindness.

I remember how utterly horrified I felt when I read this

turn of events. I felt sick for this young girl and the cruel fate that was hers. Laura recounts in later books how she walked with Mary on the vast prairies surrounding their various homes and described to her older sister how the prairie grass waved and undulated like water. During those walks she was Mary's eyes. And now here I was with Neil, and Laura was my mentor, and I couldn't help but wonder why it was that this event in this book had affected me so deeply and stayed with me for so many years.

*n*AS LONG AS I LIVE I'LL remember the outings with my mother as she pushed me in my wheelchair through the suburban neighborhoods surrounding the rehab center. Reliving it and recounting it today causes a lump to form in my throat. She weighs about one hundred and twenty pounds when she's wet and wearing boots, yet she deftly maneuvered me and my formidable chair down the winter-worn sidewalks, many cracked and uneven from February's frost heaves.

Getting out of the hospital for some fresh air and a change of scene—to rejoin the world again—was part of out daily routine, one we both looked forward to. And we went with the blessing of the rehab hospital staff. Sometimes Mom and I talked the whole time—we were easy in each other's company. We covered topics from the meditation class she had signed up for to the progress I was making in physical therapy. Other times we maintained a peaceful silence, focusing on our own sense experiences. Winter was on its way out, giving way to the smells and sounds of spring's return at last.

I don't remember our speaking directly about my blindness. I think it was too hard for either of us to talk about. It was still fresh and raw and early in the transition from what had been to what lay ahead. It was still surreal, and I think we both, in the back of our minds, were hoping that my sight would somehow miraculously be restored. We were still within the window of time that it could possibly, however remotely, happen. Or maybe we just didn't want to go there—didn't want to tarnish a positive part of our day. But talking or silent, being direct or keeping our own council, the bond that formed between us was a gift I cherished then and still do.

*a*MIA'S BIRTHDAY WAS IN MID-MARCH, just four days after Neil's. Neil and I decided, the day before her birthday, to go for our usual walk and before returning to his room stop at the hospital gift shop and choose a present that he could give her the next day.

"Yay," I thought, "We have a plan, a purpose, a normal activity that normal people do. We're kind of like normal people." But the new normal completely unhinged us.

I had scouted out the gift shop on my own prior to our outing and had been impressed with its quality. There were lots of unique items, and the jewelry was unusually creative for a hospital gift shop. I knew we'd find something Mia would like.

She was a jewelry person, like me, and Neil had enjoyed, in the past, buying earrings for both of us for special occasions.

We entered the shop after our walk, and I maneuvered Neil's wheelchair to the jewelry section. I took a pair of earrings off the rack and placed them in his hands so he could feel their shape, their length, their weight. At the same time, I described them—the design, the color, what about them stood out. Neil hesitated, seemed unsure. I grabbed a second pair and went through the same process of trying to make use of his tactile sense in conjunction with the auditory that I could provide. Wanting him to have some choice—after all the gift was from him, not from me—we went through the tedious process several more times. I could see that this was not fun for him. It was totally sad, and it was frustrating.

Finally, he chose a pair and we got in line behind another person who was making a purchase. And all of a sudden, Neil began to sob. I turned to him, taken aback by his expression of overwhelming grief. It took me by complete surprise, and, on the other hand, of course, it didn't. We had just lived through ten minutes of the most unendurable pain. Neil's words brought me to my knees, both literally and figuratively—"I can't even buy my girlfriend a goddamn birthday present!"

The shopper in front of us paid and left. It was our turn. But the tears streamed down my face, and as the shop keeper waited in respectful silence, I knelt down to Neil in his wheelchair, laid my head on his shoulder, and the two of us wept noisily into each others arms. What a sad vignette it must have been for anyone passing by—a display of the most extreme anguish and defeat: a thin young guy with dark glasses in a wheel chair and a little middle-aged woman clinging to each other and obviously not coping well with the life they got.

*n*IT WAS MARCH THIRTEENTH, 2008—two days after my twenty-ninth birthday and two days before Mia's. Mom and I were on a mission. After our wheelchair walk along one of our regular routes, we were going to stop by the Southside Medical Center gift shop to buy a birthday present for Mia.

Mia loved jewelry, like Mom. In true form, my mother had checked out the gift shop in short order after arriving here. She told me that the earrings in the shop were awesome, a definite cut above the usual hospital gift shop merchandise.

I wanted to get something special for Mia, something beautiful, something that in some small way would show my eternal gratitude for all she had done, not only for me but for all of us. This mission, this plan, was a small and simple one. I'd been a pretty decisive guy in my former life. Deliberation and indecision were not personal traits that tripped me up or caused me unnecessary angst.

But that guy was gone—or at least major, defining parts of him were gone. And around every corner I had to confront a new, diminished, broken guy with pathetic limitations. And I had to move into that guy's skin, feel like a foreigner, and somehow learn to accept him—like him—be him. And that was no easy feat.

We entered the gift shop, bringing the brisk March air in with us. Mom seemed to mean business as she pushed me down an aisle and parked me where she had planned—in front of a small, wire rack of silver and stone jewelry. I could hear her rotating the rack and heard the tinkle as delicate beads and wires swayed with the motion.

My mother placed a pair of earrings attached to a small square of cardboard in my hands. And she started in on her newly developing skill of describing details. She took my index finger and moved it along the length of one of the earrings in a valiant yet futile attempt to have me feel the beauty that I could not see.

All of a sudden, the space I was inhabiting began to shrink. It felt like walls were closing in on me, ready to squeeze the breath out of my body. I couldn't feel anything I was touching. I couldn't feel anything at all. How could I pick out something for Mia with my groping index finger alone? Without ever getting to see it? I felt like I was bringing nothing to the table. All I could do was nod my head in agreement as I held each potential gift, pretending to feel and understand the dainty craftsmanship.

The undeniable heartbreak of my situation finally caught up with me that afternoon in the hospital gift shop, and after weeks of maintaining a fake stoicism, I finally fell apart. My mother and I have always operated in tandem when it comes to emotions, and the sadness of the situation was not lost on her. She watched me disintegrate before her eyes, and it was too much to endure: my break-down became her break-down. We held each other in a tight embrace, both sobbing as we waited in line to pay for the earrings we'd randomly selected. Our shoulders heaved in unison without self-consciousness or shame for our socially awkward behavior. All my sorrow—all my tears for Mia, my family, my beloved students at Greenwood, everything I'd lost—fell onto my mother's neck and shoulders.

When we finally gained enough composure to pay for the gift that, in all honesty, my mother selected by herself, the cashier responded to us with simple compassion. She asked no questions, offered no sympathy. The gift she gave us that afternoon was respectful patience, even in the presence of others waiting in line behind us. And Mom and I agreed, as we made our way upstairs to my room, that even tiny, unheralded gifts, like the one she had given us, qualified you as an angel.

ONE DAY WE GOT A MESSAGE from the nurses' station that the director of Vermont Division for the Blind, Joe Stein, was dropping by to meet Neil. He wanted to assess Neil's condition and needs, tell him about services available and, basically, welcome us into the world of blindness, I guess. He knew that Neil would be returning home very soon and that we were going to need help.

Early in the afternoon a man appeared at the door—the thinnest man I had ever met. He had a reserved demeanor, a little shy even, but with a friendly, open face. Something about him put me at ease. Later we would learn that Joe, himself, was a cancer survivor who needed, permanently, to be on a very restricted diet. Because of his own background, Joe understood our stress regarding Neil's health. He also understood that Neil would be learning how to how to deal with his blindness at the same time that he was taking radiation and chemotherapy—a pretty tall order.

That first time meeting Joe was difficult, to say the least. I can see him standing at the foot of Neil's bed, Neil's occupational therapist and a couple nurses gathered round so he could demonstrate to them and to us how one does "sighted guide" with a blind person. The image of Joe and the assembled audience is seared so deeply within me because it was a cruel smack of reality that threatened the protective shell I had built around myself—the shell that encased my hope that Neil's sight would miraculously be restored. While the memory of Joe's visit that afternoon is visually strong for me, it remains a confusing blur regarding my receiving any of the information he presented. I was so overwhelmed by the newness of Neil's situation that I was unable to hear much of what he said. Only sinister words and phrases come to mind now: white cane, mobility instruction, life skills, braille, transportation issues. Thankfully, Jim seemed to be maintaining a steady presence, and I knew he could fill me in later when a channel might open in my brain and I could process information like a normally functioning person.

As it turned out, I needed Jim's resolute presence right then and there. For as I looked over at Neil I could see that he had become a shell. He just wasn't there. He had withdrawn to some place very deep within in an effort to protect himself from what he was hearing, from the future that was being spelled out. But he did speak up in the end—he did respond—and this is what he said: "I'm not going to need what you're telling me about because I'm not going to be blind."

Jim told him gently that we had not abandoned hope—that things could still change, improve. Joe may well have encountered this kind of denial before as he was quick to explain that his job was to meet the needs of any Vermonter experiencing vision loss even if the situation proved to be temporary. We made plans with Joe to meet again once Neil left the hospital and was settled in at home. And, in the end, Joe Stein and Vermont Division for the Blind played an essential, supportive role in Neil's new life.

Following Joe's visit, Neil fell into one of his long, deep sleeps. Like always, I prayed that it served the healing of his body and his brain. But that day I asked for more—that it serve as powerful medicine for an overloaded mind and sorrow as deep as a well.

*W*WHILE I LINGERED IN A DEEP state of denial about my blindness, the wheels of life continued to spin. One morning a man entered my room at Southside. He greeted me in a quiet, almost gentle voice. He seemed polite and maybe a little formal. He introduced himself as Joe Stein and asked if he could speak with me. The moment I said "Yes" I heard a chair scraping up to my bedside. He proceeded to tell me that he worked for the Vermont Division for the Blind and Visually Impaired, and I can tell you that any intimacy I'd felt for such a friendly greeting was sucked immediately from the room. A door just slammed shut in my head. He was the last person I wanted to see or, more accurately, talk to. I wished I could change my mind about inviting him in. Apparently, word that I had lost my sight was now common knowledge, and it had fallen upon the appropriate ears of the agency that works with blind Vermonters. So they sent one of their minions to make contact with me.

I didn't want to hear whatever message or information he came to relay. Every time I heard the word "blind" I would cringe. I didn't want to be force fed information about services available to me—life skills, mobility training, technology lessons. All I heard was that one horrible word repeating and echoing again and again inside my head, and it made me feel sick to my stomach. I was incapable of taking in anything this Joe Stein might have said. Not only was I in denial, I was probably rude due to my depression regarding my state.

Looking back on the situation, I would say Joe deserved a raise or at least some kind of official social work award or honor just for dealing with me that day. He remained calm and resilient in the face of the blank mask I must have displayed. Internally, I was furious. Was my family completely resigned to the fact that they now had a blind son—a handicapped family member? Because I never would be. This was surely a temporary state. So I ignored everything Joe said and offered no response. I simply wanted to be left alone. Despite my best efforts, however, a completely unbroken, totally supportive, and maddeningly understanding Joe Stein took his leave, telling me he would see me again when I returned home so we could set up a schedule of support services.

*a*I HAD BEEN ATTENDING THE WEEKLY staff meetings at Southside to listen to the reports from the team of therapists who worked with Neil. They were happy to have family members be part of the team as well as the patients, themselves. I felt as though I had my finger on the pulse of all that was happening with Neil, so I was completely brought up short, as I had been at University-North, when the director of the Southside rehab wing announced that Neil was ready to be released and that the date was just around the corner.

"How could this be," I thought, my mind reeling at the prospect of Neil's therapy sessions and support being so suddenly withdrawn. And then it dawned on me—the "hidden agenda," the "ah-ha" realization—that this decision had been made by the insurance company. Its support was surely coming to its predetermined end and that was the driving factor. When I asked this question, the director admitted that my hunch was true.

"But what you must keep in mind," he explained, "is that insurance companies make their determinations based on the regular reports they receive from the professionals who work with a patient. Based on Neil's progress, it's been determined that the services he's received have been successful. The goals have been met."

I did, however, learn something else that afternoon. Part of a rehab hospital's job is to determine if the setting to which the patient is being released is equipped to meet his or her needs for accommodation. And based on that, we did, in the end, buy a few extra days at Southside. Neil would be moving in with Jim and me, into the house he had grown up in, for the duration of his six weeks of radiation and year of chemotherapy. He would reside in the largest bedroom of the house which had its own small bathroom. The shower stall in that bathroom was antiquated and rusty and needed to be replaced. The project required some carpentry, and Jim was at home, racing to complete the job. When it was finished it would be the perfect accommodation for Neil—no tub to step over and a shower space that was small enough that he could never fall and hurt himself if he should lose his balance. There would always be a wall to catch him and keep him upright. The staff was very pleased to hear about the bathroom and had no problem procuring a later discharge date for him.

And that was that. We did arrange prior to his discharge for Neil to become a patient in the outpatient PT department for a couple of weeks. He had just started using a white cane, and we felt that more mobility practice and some balance work would be worth paying for out-of-pocket. This plan buoyed me up some in that it provided a plan and a schedule for our very first days at home after two months in hospital settings. We could get up in the morning and have a clear purpose, someone waiting for us.

Our next stage in this arduous journey was about to begin. On the day of Neil's release, as the nurses and therapists lined up to hug him good-bye and to wish us well, I breathed a silent prayer for him and for us—a prayer for the strength to navigate the long days ahead, one step at a time, for faith that things could and would get better, and for the ability to make the best of this new and unfamiliar life.

*n*THE DAY I LEFT SOUTHSIDE was emotional for me. Not only was I leaving my den with its predictable rhythms and schedules, feeding times and interactions, to re-enter the real world as a completely different person, I was leaving my pack of female healers—a huge support in my life. I think they were sad to bid me farewell as well. I knew my appreciation of their special talents as well as my youthful spunk had been a gift—the only kind I could have offered. I was sure they would miss my non-stop flirting and garbled, horrendous excuses for it: "Hey I was just practicing my speech!" I had blossomed under each of their care, had made undeniable progress that they could be proud of.

We were in a tight group giving good-bye hugs and last words of wisdom and all that. Despite the cacophony of voices I heard a familiar female voice saying, "Neil?" with a kind of question mark at the end of "Neil." I recognized it as Ellie's. I turned in the direction of her voice. She asked me, quietly, if she could give me a good-bye hug. I started to laugh—after all we had been through together—the countless showers, teeth brushing, deodorant application, locating the damn toilet, and she needed my permission for a simple hug? It just shows how much of an angel Ellie is.

I said, "Ellie, you've been helping me shower for the last three weeks. It's because of you that my weak, naked body didn't just topple over. Get over here!" And I gave her the biggest, deepest, most grateful hug I had in me.

~

You may be thinking as you read this account from my rehab days that I am an unusually upbeat guy despite all the horrible things I'd gone through to that point. That may have appeared to be true, but it was by no means the whole story. Deep within, I lived in a state of despair that I tried to exercise my way out of. While on the outside I was the most vivacious, most enthusiastic patient who'd ever sucked on a button or worked an exercise machine, I knew the truth—nothing was going to put it off forever. No matter how many buttons I pushed around in my mouth or how many stairs I climbed, nothing was going to change that truth. The cold hard fact was that I suffered from a life-threatening brain tumor and if that, in itself, didn't plunge me into a dark place, the loss of my vision most certainly did.

EVEN BEFORE NEIL AND I SWUNG out of the parking lot of Southside Medical Center and headed west for Vermont, I said, "Let's go out to lunch to celebrate your homecoming. This is a real milestone for you."

I was determined to be out in the world, doing everyday

things, leading as regular a life as we could, and I figured we might as well start on Day One of being released from eight weeks of hospital living. Neil was game. We decided to go to our favorite Chinese restaurant, Panda North, in Brattleboro. On the way we planned what we would order, given that Neil was still a novice at chewing and swallowing solid food. Many of the things we liked there were moist and slippery, not that we had ever categorized them that way before, but our new, unfamiliar life required new considerations. We decided that a noodle dish, Szechuan dumplings, and soup were the right choice for us. Perfect for a rookie swallower.

As we made our way from the car to the front door of the restaurant, I realized that this, too, was a first. We had not walked together outdoors or into a public place. Neil had his white cane in hand but leaned heavily on me, his balance still unsteady. I had his arm folded in mine and kept it close to my body, and in this way I "steered" him. I still didn't quite understand how "sighted guide" worked, and Neil still needed more physical support than he would in the days to come.

As we followed our waitress down an aisle to our table, I heard my name being called. Seated at a table we were passing were my two meditation teachers, a couple who had held our family in their hearts and prayers these many weeks. I introduced them to Neil, and as we spoke briefly I thought, "Yet another first for the two of us." We were interacting with people who knew Neil's story and now could see his brand new way of being in the world. Suddenly I felt exhausted. It felt like a lifetime of "firsts" lay ahead.

When I recall that first meal out together, I think of it as successful, but not pleasurable. In truth, it was more like a test we passed than a special treat. To our credit, we did it, but it was such hard work. Eating was still not natural or automatic for Neil. He had to concentrate on every bite, focusing single-mindedly on both the chewing and swallowing. The other issue he had not yet learned to handle was the fact that the left side of his mouth did not work like his normally functioning right side. Food would get stuck in the stationary side, against his inner cheek, and he would have to manually move it with his finger in order to swallow it. Needless to say, we were not yet ready for polite company, and the meal passed without us being able to speak to each other at all. Thankfully for both of us, Neil's stomach couldn't hold much food, and we ended up taking the remainder home for Jim.

*n*AFTER HEARTFELT GOOD-BYES AND good-lucks from those who had helped me and cared about me at Southside, we crossed what felt like an endless parking lot at a snail's pace. I had not yet gained mastery of the walker I was leaving the hospital with. It shimmied and bounced in front of me under the uneven pressure of my weak arms.

Once I was seated in the passenger side of my mom's car, she leaned over and located the seat belt for me. I felt like a decrepit old man. I promised myself that I would learn to do things on my own as soon as possible, but I certainly wasn't there yet. Without my vision, the simplest things seemed complicated. But despite all the negative thoughts swirling within me, I reminded myself that this was a happy day. I was being released from the hospital at long last, and I could swallow on my own. All my progress, the baby steps and the giant steps, were cause for celebration. As we headed toward Vermont, Mom suggested that to celebrate we go to lunch at Panda North, one of my favorite restaurants. "Right on," I responded. "This will be my first full meal, minus the aftertaste of barium!"

As we were shown to our table and I felt for my seat, it struck me that this was the real deal—I was actually going to be eating out! For months as I lay in the darkness in hospital rooms with tubes in just about every orifice, I had fantasized about the feasts I would have someday. But caution had prevailed, and before our arrival Mom and I had planned what we would order from a menu I knew pretty well. We had foresight enough to be conservative and not overly-ambitious with our choices. We had reviewed things that did not take a lot of chewing and were easy to swallow. I had decided on two of my old-time favorites, both so moist they may as well have been predigested—hot and sour soup and Szechuan dumplings.

Before the food arrived I felt a hint of anxiety and vulnerability that would accompany the many "firsts" that lay ahead of me: was I even ready for restaurant dining? Before I could work myself up over this question, however, the food arrived.Forget chopsticks—each bite was proceeded by several fruitless stabs of my fork before I could capture a slimy little szechuan dumpling on the tines. Chewing it, as soft as it was, took more effort than I had anticipated.

The food itself felt like a whole new experience. Everything tasted so much more overwhelming than I expected. I was shocked at how intensely strong all of the flavors were. Each morsel that I successfully aimed into my mouth was full of competing tastes. The dumplings, which swam around in my once loved peanut sauce, were exceedingly sweet, yet, at the same time, they were quite salty—almost too salty. The hot and sour soup, which I had formerly believed was neither of the two, tasted exactly as its name implied. The spices in the broth tasted so foreign to my palate it made my throat tighten up and my mouth and the left side of my face reflexively cringe, like I had just bitten down on a lemon. In addition, during their prolonged hiatus from eating, my lips and tongue had grown hyper-sensitive to heat. Each little spoonful of soup I brought to my lips felt scalding. I had eaten at this restaurant countless times before, and I cannot recall the soup being so astonishingly hot. What I did remember is that I used to tease Mia as she blew on each spoonful before she put it in her mouth. I'd call her "Tender Lips." Now it was me who recoiled from its temperature. By the end of the meal I was exhausted.

It would have been a real stretch for any onlookers to recognize our presence at Panda North that day as a celebration, as not a word was exchanged between my mother and me throughout the entire ordeal. After the fact, I have to say that no one I know would have had the gumption or the optimism to take me straight from rehab to a Chinese restaurant except for my incredible mother. Maybe it was my imagination, tinged with a bit of paranoia, but I thought I heard out of the corner of my good ear, from the lips of a little kid at a nearby table—"Look at that man, Mommy—is he eating?" I can't be a visual witness, but I am sure my mom kept her chin high as she quietly moved my napkin under my hand, just to remind me it was there.

After this vigorous workout—filling my stomach the old fashioned way—we made our way back to the car and I was once again strapped into my seat belt. Now I felt less like a decrepit old man and more like an enormous baby boy, which was no less demeaning. Despite feeling so low about who I now seemed to be, I properly played the part and fell fast asleep for the remaining half hour trip home.

My mother pulled into our driveway and cut off the engine. Here we were at the old house I had grown up in, my eyes still tightly closed. But there was no question in my mind that we were in the middle of the quiet, quaint village of Westminster West.

Mom reached over and gently shook me back into the dark reality of my life—a life in which I was perpetually a Beginner, a Novice. Part of me wished I could just remain seated in the car forever with my eyes closed. But I responded, reaching for where I guessed the door lever might be. This fumbling hunt opened the door to the beginning of my new life.

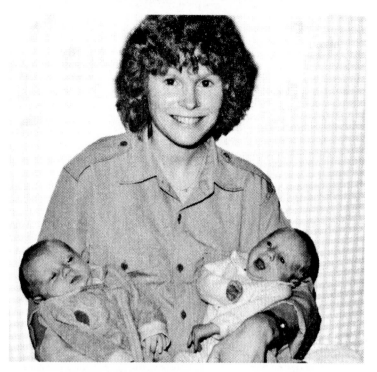

Our fraternal twin boys were born in March 1979. How were we so lucky to get both of them at once?

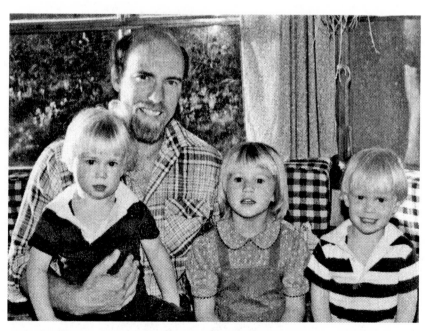

Jim and our young family pose on Jessica's first day of kindergarten.

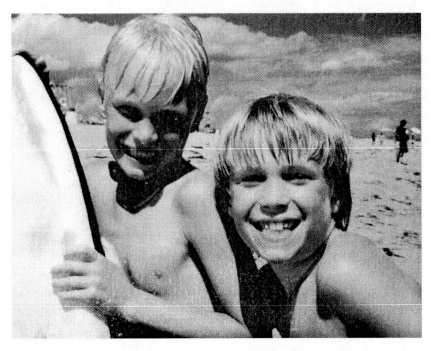

Neil and Jackson on our annual summer vacation to the Rhode Island shore.

Skateboarding at the
University of Redlands,
Redlands, California

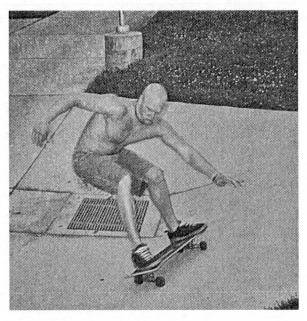

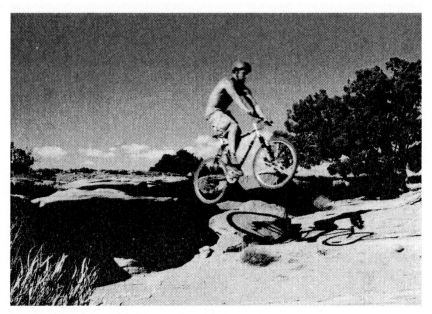

Above: Mountain biking in Salt Lake City, Utah.

Below: Exercise, including body building, has supported Neil through thick and thin.

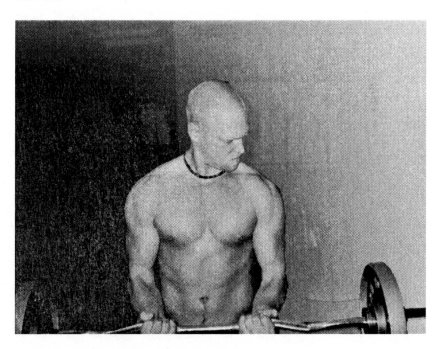

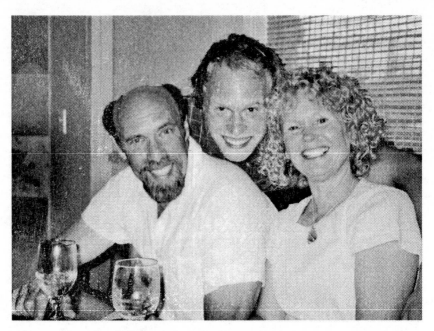

Above: Celebrating Neil's graduation from college in May 2002

Below: This is the last photo of our three children before Neil's surgery and blindness. We were together for Christmas in 2007. Neil confided in his brother and sister that he feared he might have a brain tumor.

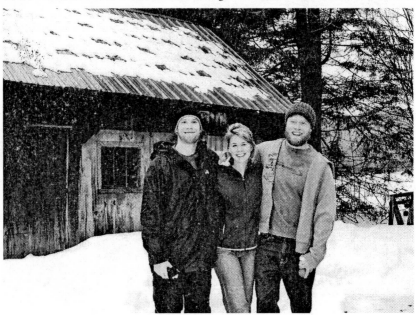

PART TWO

A Full Year

SIX

A YEAR OF HEALING

Let go of the way you thought life
would unfold; the holding of plans
or dreams or expectations. Let it
all go. Save your strength to swim
with the tide. Take this on faith:
the mind may never find the
explanations that it seeks, but
you will move forward, nonetheless.

~ Danna Faulds

NEIL AND JIM AND I BECAME housemates from the spring of 2008 until the end of August 2009. There was never a day in that chapter of our lives that didn't hold a measure of grief and disbelief for me about what had happened to Neil, of fear that a happy life for him was an impossibility, of crushing responsibility for both Jim and me to serve as anchors, beacons of hope, cheerleaders whose job was to elicit optimism. Neil had completely lost his independence—could do nothing on his own beyond his personal care and the navigation of our home, which, with practice, he learned fairly quickly. With prompting from us he began to "see" in his mind's eye the layout of the house in which he'd grown up. He would never have that advantage again in any other space he would inhabit or visit, so we considered ourselves lucky. But no longer could he jump in the car and do an errand, toss a lacrosse ball with Jim and Jackson in the yard, run down the road on his own to visit a neighbor, open the refrigerator door, size up the contents, and grab what looked good, get up in the morning and head to the job he'd loved. The losses were staggering.

*n*SO HERE I WAS, BACK IN the home where I'd grown up. Two major hospitals in northern New England had had their way with me, chewed me up and spit me out into the spittoon that my life had become. I had gone to sleep in a hospital, interrupting my busy and happy existence, to wake up to nothing. The life that had been mine, that I had forged with so much trial and error, was not my life anymore.

There were all kinds of reasons to be grateful for no longer being held in the medicinal clutches of those hospitals. Gone was the foreign, antiseptic smell accompanying each breath I took, the patient down the hall coughing throughout the night, nurses whispering my vital signs to their replacements at shift-change time.

But, at the same time, I no longer had an array of friendly, encouraging professionals to help me through each day. My parents' home was bereft of personal trainers to cheer on my stair-stepping prowess. I no longer had a speech pathologist to impress with my remarkable progress. My time had come and gone. I was no longer the hero of the neurology ward or the bad boy of rehab. And it was hard to pick through the scraps of my former life in an attempt to build some kind of new one.

I continued to have angst-filled dreams based on my former life as teacher, coach, and dorm head at the Greenwood School. It would take a few minutes of agitated confusion in the middle of the night before it dawned on me, yet again, that the boys were gone to me, no longer relied on or needed me. That was finished.

As I lay in darkness, my mind would wander into dangerous places. I still had hope that if I tried hard enough, at least a fraction of my sight would slowly return. If I could find just one little spot in my otherwise entirely black field of vision, I would work with it as I had worked on every other area of weakness I had struggled with. I would have enormous patience if I could simply locate a point where I could make out a vague shadow, the outline of a shape, a blurry light. I would focus all my effort on this small sign of hope because it would have the potential to grow in size and clarity. I had to rely on this possibility to soften the fact that nearly everything in my life that had sustained me and given me pleasure had turned to ash.

NOW AND THEN, DURING THOSE early days, I would close my eyes to imagine what it might feel like to be Neil. And I would want to scream at the horror of it. I felt as though I couldn't catch my breath, that I was drowning. The only thing that made me feel worse was opening my eyes again, putting an end to the frightening game of pretend while knowing that for Neil, so lovable, so good, that was never an option.

One sunny spring afternoon, I emerged from my bedroom where I had been resting. I heard Neil stirring in his room, preparing, I figured, to come downstairs following his afternoon nap. I waited for him, but he didn't emerge. When I peeked into the room, I saw that he was still in the bed, curled in a fetal position with his back toward me. Had I been wrong? Was he still asleep? I tiptoed toward the bed and said his name. He turned toward me. His cheeks were wet and his face distorted in pain. "It's not fair," he sobbed, "It's just not fair."

I froze. I was taken completely by surprise, and in the next instant I could feel the actual physical sensation, once again, of my heart breaking. I leaned down and held him in my arms. And without effort, without any conscious forcing of my will, I went to a place outside of my own anguish to be the buoy for Neil. It is amazing what love can do. It can fill every fiber of your being with a strength, a determination, and a creativity that you could never engender by the sheer wanting of it.

I said, "Neil, get up. Come outside with me." I led him into the springtime yard, and together we felt the sun on our faces, the warm grass under our feet. We put words to the experience and we reveled in it. We explored our other senses together; the feel of a fern frond, the smell of the soil coming to life after months of dormancy. We sat by the edge of the brook—Neil's childhood playground—and listened to the springtime surge. We recalled how in late summer the water level is so low the sound is reduced to a mere trickle. We held hands and absorbed the tremendous healing that comes from being in nature and being with another human being who has shared your life and will always be there for you. We channeled some light into the darkness of our hearts. I accepted the possibility that complete healing for us might never happen. But that afternoon we experienced soothing and the kind of peace that emerges when unbearable burdens are shouldered together.

Weeks of trauma had passed before that spring day, interminable days in the hospital and rehab center, and Neil had never once uttered the words, "It's not fair," or "Why me?" And he never has since that day. I had known when we named him that "Neil" is a Celtic name that means "champion." Neil is true to the name we chose for him. He has continually emerged a champion of the spirit who understands when to accept and when to strive and that a life well lived includes a measure of both.

~

A major function that Neil had left was his ability to talk, to communicate, to verbally connect, to visit. And while Neil and I had always had a strong connection, an ease of being together, similar points of view, a shared sense of humor, and common interests, there were times during those long days at home that I panicked that we would run out of material, that there would be nothing left to say. And silence was my greatest fear. During those new, raw days, optimism and cheerfulness were the only medicines I could offer. Silence felt like it surely must be, for Neil, a dark and lonely hallway of uncertainty and disorientation. He needed words as a frame of reference for what was happening or not happening. They were his only link to where I was in space and in approximation to him. If I leafed through a magazine or quietly jotted a list to take to the supermarket, Neil, of course, was left out of what was happening around him. And the only way to know what was happening was to ask.

All of a sudden, for me, the simple acts of life, the quiet, mundane routines of existence, required verbal communication, and I had to stretch myself even further than I already had. I had to practice a new way of being in the world when Neil and I were together. I started to verbally label what I was doing before he needed to inquire. This addition to my plate was due to the loss on his. Each adjustment that was required of us, each newly adopted behavior, not yet habituated, took an emotional and physical toll on both of us and led to fatigue.

Yes, I had my frustrations, but more than anything I feared that this new reality was too overwhelming, and that Neil would give up. I dreaded the possibility of him turning to me and proclaiming, "Hey—the life I got just ain't worth all this effort." What if the pit of despair, its gaping mouth always hungry, just sucked him in? Would it be, in the end, just too damn hard to resist, to fight, to win?

~

I began to rely on alcohol at the end of each day. I had always enjoyed a five o'clock beer or two several times a week. But alcohol now became a mecca of escapism for me, a tempting, temporary release from the grinding responsibility I felt and a salve for the despair that stalked me. During the summer of 2008, I'd sit in the kitchen with a micro-brew in my hand. I can see myself very clearly on a particular early evening—a snapshot of many other evenings. Neil is out having dinner with a friend, one of the angels who is standing by him and supporting him. Jim and Jessica are making dinner together. I sit. And as I sit and sip, I begin to weep. My body sags in defeat, my head sinks low. It's waterworks time. Jim and Jessica say nothing. Engaging with me would be fruitless. They just keep working on dinner. Silently, nursing their own sadness, they move around me. My tears flow as we sit and eat together. They are just part of everything in our awful life.

∼

Following his release from rehab, I remained at home with Neil for three weeks before returning to my teaching job toward the end of April. I was very anxious about resuming my duties in a world I was no longer used to, about leaving my newly blind son alone for most of the day. My world had become a cocoon. I was reluctant to emerge and have to deal with people. My feelings were those of a new mother facing the end of maternity leave. I was nervous, uncertain, and guilty about leaving the nest I had built for my baby and me.

But these were my own feelings; they were never verbalized by Neil who encouraged me to claim my life, even as he was striving to build his own. If he had reservations about being on his own for hours, if he feared feeling lonely, sad, or isolated, he kept his own council. Perhaps he had no idea what it would feel like. Or maybe he was ready, willing, even eager to attempt a portion of his life on his own. Jim was clear that I needed to go back to my job, that I must, and that it would be good for both Neil and me. I believed him, but I had to do it on my own terms, slowly.

I made an appointment with my principal in order to work out a plan of reentry into the classroom that no longer felt like mine. I arrived at school to find that he was still busy with another matter. I would have to wait a bit. I sat on the bench outside the office amid a flow of children, parents, and staff coming and going about their various business. I was thinner than I'd been ten weeks earlier, and I wore dark glasses. I needed the glasses as a filter from the world's hubbub, its glare. In my mind, they provided me a little distance and some protection from intrusion. I felt vulnerable and removed from the person I had been. If the dark glasses made me seem somewhat unapproachable, that was fine with me.

The school counselor, whom I'd always liked, happened by. He plunked down on the bench next to me, gave me a hug, and engaged me in a warm and caring conversation. I did just fine—my outward behavior, my responses were totally appropriate—but why was it that I felt strangely removed? I was like a small island, separate and remote.

The meeting with my principal went well. He was happy to see me after so many weeks and was supportive of the plan I proposed. I asked to return to my classroom following April vacation and work three days a week through the month of May, sharing the job with the young woman who had taken over in my absence. I hoped to work Monday through Wednesday and have her cover Thursdays and Fridays. We would co-teach in this manner for six weeks until Jessica arrived in Vermont on June first for the summer. With Jessica at home to support Neil, I felt I'd be able to finish the school year full time. I could reclaim my position, my confidence, and end the school year like I would begin it in September, fully present, fully in charge.

My principal felt the plan was a good one with one addition of his own. The week I started back he wanted my replacement to be present as well, overlapping my three days. He needed to do what was best for the children. I had evaporated from their lives on the last day of January. Now it was mid-April. It had been unsettling for all of them and traumatic for some at their tender age. He didn't want a similar grieving to happen by disrupting their routine with their new teacher.

I understood completely and agreed with him. I left feeling happy. I was taking a step forward, a step toward resuming a life that I had inhabited, a life that had been mine. Nothing in my life would ever really be the same, but there were parts I could reclaim with the hope that they would ground me, support me, heal me.

～

During the summer of 2008, Joe Stein from Vermont Division for the Blind began making home visits regularly. He was a calm and steady presence, compassionate regarding our grief and matter-of-fact in describing services offered by the state, most of which would be conducted in our home. He was ready to begin the process of scheduling the personnel who would begin teaching Neil how to adapt to his new existence. Neil could be offered lessons in beginning Braille, mobility training, life skills, and computer training. Joe explained that he was required to write a formal plan, with specific goals in these various areas. He would monitor Neil's progress at regular intervals. He also cautioned us to keep the big picture in mind: Neil would be undergoing treatment for his cancer in the months ahead. The treatment would likely compromise his energy somewhat, although he had a hunch that Neil's age and prior fitness were assets that would serve him well in tolerating the six weeks of radiation and the twelve cycles of chemotherapy.

While I appreciated Joe's counsel and respected his experience as a cancer survivor, I glossed over his advice to move ahead with caution and deliberation. I could not have explained, or perhaps even recognized at the time, that what was keeping me afloat was purposeful activity, plans, a sense of moving forward. This way of being was essential to my sanity. In two months time I would be returning to my classroom again and Jessica would be returning to North Carolina. What I needed for my own well-being, as well as for Neil's, was absolute assurance that when Neil was on his own all day, he would be living as full and fulfilling a life as possible.

Jessica and I were already brainstorming possible activities that would enrich Neil's life in the year ahead. Neil in no way put the brakes on the possibilities we presented. He seemed every bit as eager to move ahead as he had been in the rehab gym. His desire was to sign up for all the services Joe could provide and intersperse them with several other activities. The three of us began to put together a calendar that would shape the days and weeks of Neil's upcoming year.

We agreed that Neil should have at least one scheduled activity each day while he was alone. In addition, each day would include ample time for a nap and free time to make phone calls, listen to books on tape as well as to National Public Radio news. These were all things that Neil proposed and wanted to do. Not only would they fill his time, they would make him, as he said, a better person, not just a better blind person.

Joe admitted that he had not seen a family rally so fast after a member's sudden and traumatic loss of vision. I'm sure our intensity was not lost on him. Whether he was impressed by us or thought our vision unrealistic, taking on too much too soon, pushing too hard, he was ever supportive.

∼

Neil and I talked about the benefit of his seeing a therapist in order to process the trauma he'd endured and the unknowns that lay ahead. He agreed. His new reality was still hard to grasp, let alone to bear. He needed guidance in dealing with his immense grief and his fears of living with a life-threatening illness. My own therapist recommended a young colleague she thought would be a great match for Neil, and, indeed, the two of them bonded from their first session. Their schedule of appointments became a priority on Neil's calendar.

n I AM A SENSITIVE GUY; I'M NOT afraid to admit it. And that's why I agreed with Mom right off that anyone who had gone through all that I had, who had lost so much and who needed help envisioning what the future would bring, would benefit from seeing a therapist. I'd heard from others that it can take a couple of tries to find the right match, but I lucked out immediately. Through some networking, Mom got the name of a therapist who was not much older than I was but who'd had a well established practice for some time.

Appointments with Erica became a mainstay on my calendar the year I lived with my parents, and Erica became a lifeline for me. She was the person I could pour my heart out to, could cry in front of, could talk with about any topic I wanted or needed to, totally uncensored. My way of being in her office was private, of course, and clearly separated from my daily life. She was so open and made me feel that not only did she understand my grief, she felt it as well. And that was really important to me.

Sometimes after a particularly sad session, a session in which I had broken down and cried, a change would occur deep inside me. It was as though I'd been wrung out, but in a good way, and I would feel so much better. Now the word "catharsis" had personal meaning to me. Our appointments gave me the opportunity to face my emotions and work with them, not ignore or gloss over them. And I just couldn't do this kind of processing with my family. We were all trying to keep our heads above water, and the last thing I wanted to do was increase their sorrow. I wanted to protect them from that. But my emotions would bottle up inside me and I needed a venue to let them out. I had no worries about making Erica sad because this was her job, and she was great at it.

～

Although the work on my inner being was new to me, the rehabilitation of my outer being, my physical body, was not a new endeavor. There was no question in my mind that the restoration of my physical health and well-being was as important as my mental/emotional health.

Ever since I was a pipsqueak, I'd always loved to work out, had been enamored with the idea of lifting weights to make myself stronger and more muscular. My heroes were the old bodybuilders, Arnold Schwarzenegger, Franco Colombo, and Lou Ferrigno, and I must have watched an old VHS copy of *Pumping Iron* a thousand times. While my father, my brother, and I work out religiously today, I was the debut weight lifter in the family. I would close the doors of our front room where my dad had installed a cheap Weider bench set complete with old-school sand filled plastic weights. Motivated by how scrawny I was, especially compared to my seemingly enormous father, I would tirelessly work out by myself until I was dripping with sweat. In retrospect, I was doing everything wrong, with poor form and an overambitious weight selection, but it didn't matter because I thought it was the coolest thing I'd ever done. I swore I could feel my pipe cleaner-sized arms grow bigger with every workout. It was just a matter of time before I could compete with my bodybuilding heroes. I'm sure my parents were somewhat bewildered that my bedroom walls were plastered with posters of grotesquely steroid-induced bodybuilders.

Following my brain surgery I have my father to thank for helping me get my weakened body back in shape. By the time I was released from rehab, the old sand weights were long gone, replaced by a solid lifting machine my father, brother, and I had bought years ago when Jackson and I were teenagers. That machine had become our temple of fitness back then and now would play a huge role in my physical rehabilitation.

Dad and I agreed that we should take it super easy for my first workout which occurred one day after being released from rehab. Although I had been working out under the tutelage of Gail in the rehab gym at Southside, I hadn't been doing any lifting at all. My father watched me like a hawk that afternoon as we performed a single set of the most basic exercises. I could hardly believe that I had become so weak in a little over two months. My muscles had completely atrophied. Dad very reluctantly changed the weights from ten to twenty pounds only after I kept whining that I could and wanted to do more. Therefore, I take full respon-sibility and can only blame my overzealous pride for the results that humbled me the next morning. I could barely get out of bed. My thighs and calves quivered beneath me on the three foot trip from my bed to the bathroom. I stumbled into the shower and was more grateful than I ever thought I would be for the handles my father had installed into the tiny shower stall. They were the only reason I managed to stay upright. Dad, of course, felt guilty and responsible for my crippled state, but things started looking up after the hot shower and my mother's call to University-North for assurance that taking some ibuprofen was perfectly OK.

In keeping with the long line of "firsts" that presented more formidable challenges than I anticipated, this first workout on the weight machine was humbling. I didn't, however, let it dampen my spirit for long. I actually celebrate it as the segue for the workouts I shared with my father that year and am convinced that each one helped to stabilize my mental health just as surely as it benefited my physical health. It was with my dad that I slowly but with great determination built my physical self back to the form that felt like the "me" I had known and liked. So, thanks, mi padre, for every workout we both grunted and sweated as well as laughed our way through the year we were housemates.

*a*ONE OF THE MOST SIGNIFICANT endeavors of Neil's full year of treatment and recovery was a one-of-a-kind study of massage therapy with a generous and open-minded local practitioner. The experience of receiving a massage just prior to his surgery had so moved him, had so imprinted itself on his psyche, that he proclaimed that he, himself, wanted to become a massage therapist.

The first time I heard of his intention we were having ice cream at an outdoor cafe. We'd struck up a conversation with strangers who happened to be sitting next to us. Neil shared this new goal with them, offhandedly, concentrating on his melting cone as much as on the conversation, but I sensed his resolution, his conviction so palpably that I knew something important had just happened. Neil was forming a vision of a life that lay ahead, a life that belonged to a new, not fully formed person, a person who was emerging from a dark cocoon into a totally different world, a person who would succeed because he believed that starting over, changing direction, finding and making happiness were entirely possible.

We all experience moments of grace in our lives whether we call them that or not. They usually present themselves at the most unlikely times and places when we are just "being" and not striving. They are beautiful because of the element of surprise. It was at that cafe on that afternoon with those strangers that I felt grace wrap its diamond cloak around me. Having a plan for the future brightened my life. It didn't matter to me that the particulars of how Neil would actually become a massage therapist were somewhere out there in the universe, unknown to me and unrealistic at this point in time. But this point would change, and a time would come after Neil's treatment and recovery when he would start the journey toward the goal he'd proclaimed to the world.

Jessica, however, saw no need to wait. Of course Neil was not ready to embark on a formal study, enter a demanding program. But in her mind, other options were possible if one thought creatively. She hatched a bold plan and, with Mia's help, developed another activity that enriched Neil's life during his year in Westminster West.

She and Mia met with the services coordinator at a thriving holistic health clinic in our community where several massage therapists were on staff. They asked if she would approach the massage therapists to see if one would be willing to work one hour a week with a newly blinded young man with a mission of one day becoming a massage therapist. Reimbursement for that hour would come from Vermont Department of the Blind.

If we Taylors moved quickly, we learned that Joe Stein took the lead when it came to the area of vocational rehabilitation. It was a special focus for him, and he felt that funds were well spent if they paved the way for a blind individual to become as self-sustaining and independent as possible. Joe was behind the proposal with enthusiasm and support.

Of the four massage therapists asked, only one was interested in taking on this unique project in the midst of seeing her own clients. One was all we needed, and none of us could have imagined a more superb mentor than Chloe Grant became to Neil. Chloe was exactly Neil's age. She was easy going, patient, supportive, and ever thoughtful about adapting what she was trying to "show" to a person who could not see. Neil and Chloe met on Friday mornings for several months. Neil's task was to bring a friend or family member each week for the practice sessions. The prospect of being his subject, lying on a comfy massage table, and receiving hands-on attention was not a huge favor for many of us to offer, and Neil had no trouble rounding up volunteers.

At Chloe's recommendation, Neil practiced on a wide variety of body types: male/female, petite/heavy, delicate/muscled. As we subjects lay quietly, Chloe spoke to Neil about human anatomy. When she began using her hands, she had Neil place his hands on top of hers while explaining what she was doing. When he proceeded to copy her movements, she would, again, guide him with words as well as place her hands on top of his for tactile reinforcement and corrections.

From our experiences on the table those Friday mornings, Jessica and I could feel the difference between Chloe's long, smooth, deep, and confident strokes and Neil's tentative, uneven, inexperienced touch. As he practiced on us between lessons, we gave him honest feedback. If his pressure was too firm or not firm enough, if he unknowingly pinched our skin, we told him. He would thank us and try again. As the weeks went by, Neil's confidence and skills grew. He loved Chloe and the gift she gave him—her belief that despite his blindness he would one day enter the profession that called to him.

AFTER RESIGNING MYSELF TO THE FACT that I was blind, at least for the time being, I seized upon an idea that brought me a measure of peace and a direction to set my altered sights on: I would enter the field of massage therapy. My experience receiving a massage from John just prior to my surgery had stayed with me and affected me deeply. It had brought me undeniable tranquility at the time, and now it stood out as a ray of hope. I had been introduced to a profession with a predominantly tactile orientation, and I believed that it was the right match for me and that I would be successful. This idea, this plan, this goal became deeply embedded in me.

Chloe Grant, a local massage therapist, became my first teacher. The arrangement we had was unconventional and unique. But, then again, I, myself, was both of these things and the wonderful Chloe was as well. She was bold to take on the role of instructing me, as it was obviously uncharted territory for her, but she was ever confident and proved to be, in my estimation, a great teacher. This amazing internship came about through the out-of-the-box thinking of Jessica and Mia and was supported by Joe Stein.

My task was to provide subjects for my hour lesson for the duration of the internship. As my friends lay on the table, Chloe would describe the technique she was using, as well as its effect on the muscles, the soft tissues, even the various systems of the body. And alongside her telling, she included the showing of it by having me place my hands on top of hers. This combination was incredibly valuable to me. And we had a great time together. I was an eager student, not shy to ask questions, and Chloe seemed completely comfortable in her role as teacher. We were lit up by our common enthusiasm and our passion for this practice.

*a*BECAUSE OF NEIL'S EAGERNESS TO learn as much as he could about massage therapy, we decided that every other week he should experience massage as a client, himself. Not only would he benefit personally in terms of his own healing, helping his body withstand the effects of chemotherapy and radiation, it would provide valuable research about the profession. He would observe how a professional massage therapist conducted himself in a session and would experience the healing techniques that he was endeavoring to learn.

Neil wanted the experience of going to a male massage therapist, and he chose Ben, from the clinic where Chloe worked. Ben was a tall, affable guy who had the reputation of giving very deep, strong-pressured massages. He could offer the uniqueness of his practice and a male role model who had made this business his livelihood. Neil glowed after each session with Ben. The two of them developed a kind of brotherly camaraderie, joking and teasing each other as Ben led Neil to the massage room. They talked about life and massage while Neil was on the table and Neil reaped dual benefits: that of client and that of student. Thereafter, Neil began to practice what he was learning from Ben on those of us who supported his dream.

∼

Neil and I decided to name his full year of treatment, the twelve cycles of chemotherapy and the six weeks of radiation along with his adjustment to his new existence, the "Year of Healing." It became a mantra, a reference point for us when he sometimes lost his way and felt frustrated by the parameters of his life.

One Sunday afternoon, the two of us stood on the front porch to wave good-bye to Jackson who had driven up from

New York to spend the weekend with us. Neil felt such joy in the company of his twin brother and eagerly looked forward to Jackson's visits. Their bond was as strong as it always had been. I knew there must be a knot of pain in Jackson's heart that mirrored the pain in Jim and me. But as I watched my boys together, it seemed that not much had changed. They worked out together, teased each other as mercilessly as ever, had long conversations in the hot tub, dropped in on friends together. Without putting it into words until now, it seemed to me that Neil felt the most "whole" in the presence of his brother, that his disability was less front-and-center, less cumbersome with Jackson than with anyone else in the world. And so when Jackson would leave for home during that year, both Neil and I would go into decline. Our melancholy over missing Jackson would last a couple of days.

On this particular fall afternoon, as Neil and I stood side by side on the front porch feeling the empty space that had just held Jackson, tears welled up inside me. Neil put his arm around my shoulders: "I know why you feel sad," he said softly. "You know that you will never see me jump in my car and head off to my busy life and maybe, someday, a family. I'm not going to have those things."

"Neil," I answered, "none of us know what will happen down the line. We think we do, but we don't. There are possibilities out there that we can't even imagine. They exist for you as much as for anyone. Jackson has a job to go to, and you have one here. Your job is healing. It's not the job you chose, but it's the job before you, and you have the strength to get up every day and give it your all."

"I know, and I will," he said. And we headed inside.

~

Our focus of healing had two prongs. One had to do with trauma and loss, acceptance and readjustment. The vehicle to address this prong was our calendar of activities for the year which ultimately included beginning braille, mobility training, intermittent computer skills training, psychotherapy, massage lessons, and personal massage appointments. Each activity was either useful, pleasurable, challenging, or a combination. The activities were the building blocks of Neil's new life, and we were carefully stacking them and arranging them into the sturdy structure that would support him as he bridged who he was and who he would become.

The second prong, of course, was the physical healing of Neil's brain from cancer. In contrast to the thoughtful effort the emotional healing required, the physical strand was coming from the outside and was predetermined by the particular makeup of Neil's tumor. The first strand called for activity, the second for receptivity. That Neil's head be anchored to a table in order to receive a radiation beam to the precise area of the remaining tumor was a given. That his body be saturated with toxic chemicals which would penetrate his brain, we accepted with a grim kind of gratitude.

We were standing before a blueprint of the year that lay

ahead. As I analyzed the components of it, I felt compelled to ask myself, "Is it full? Is it responsible? Is it thorough?" In my mind I checked off the boxes for "full" and "responsible." I was satisfied. But I realized that I felt less sure, less comfortable about "thorough." If "leave no stone unturned" was etched into every fiber of my being in an effort to save my son, I could not ignore an offshoot of the healing prong, a direction we had not included in our plans: the path of faith healing.

To a northern born girl like me, faith healing had connotations of a sweltering tent somewhere in the south, the laying on of hands by a guy with big hair and a cross around his neck, and lots of swaying, swooning, and shelling out of money by gullible believers. It wasn't a world I had grown up in or been drawn to.

But between my childhood and adulthood, "alternative therapies" gained a foothold within the scientifically oriented, "attack the symptom" culture that I was most familiar with. The term "New Age" implied to me that we who live surrounded by the miracles of modern technology still have much to learn from earlier, simpler cultures that understood and made use of the gifts of the natural world. Today's offering of alternative therapies is bountiful. Some are familiar to me and many remain a mystery. But the primary goal of most, whether they be diet, body work, meditation, visualization, or healing gem stones, is the restoration of harmony and balance to our beings—mind, body and spirit. The connection of these three aspects in many cultures was a given.

Norman Cousins, who wrote *Anatomy of an Illness as Perceived by the Patient* in the seventies, came to believe that the interaction of mind, body, and spirit may impact one's health in mysterious ways. During the investigation of healing his own life-threatening illness he wrote, "Is it possible that love, hope, faith, laughter, confidence, and the will to live have positive therapeutic value?"

Living with a grim prognosis, Cousins immersed himself in studies on the effects of placebos—"pretend" drugs that have no scientific value but can sometimes yield effective results through the power of suggestion, healing patients because of their belief in their effect.

I told Neil that I very much needed him to indulge me in this area. If the two of us had agreed to label the upcoming year "The Year of Healing," we had to embrace every possibility. He was reluctant. I told him that I strongly believed in the connection between mind, spirit, and body, and how could we ignore a whole branch of healing that was gaining mainstream support because of its compelling studies and reports? He didn't feel the need for it. I had to play the only card I had left: "Neil—you have to admit that I do a lot for you. I'm asking you to do this for me."

It was a cheap shot, I admit, but he agreed. I wasn't exactly sure how a placebo could work for a dubious believer, but I had to be true to my goal of including anything and everything I thought might help, and to that end I was willing to do whatever I had to.

At the time of my request and Neil's acquiescence I had no concrete plan. I was not a strong believer in any one modality over another. My feelings were based more on intuition and the belief that there are more levels and layers to human experience than we are privy to in daily life. I found what felt to me a beautiful description of my world view sometime during this period. It is a portion of a poem called "Tomorrow's Child" by Rubin Alves:

> What is hope?
> It is the pre-sentiment that imagination
> is more real and reality is less real than it looks.
> It is the hunch that the overwhelming brutality
> of facts that oppress and repress us
> is not the last word.
> It is the suspicion that reality is more complex
> than the realists want us to believe.
> That the frontiers of the possible are not
> determined by the limits of the actual;
> and in a miraculous and unexplained way
> life is opening up creative events
> which will open the way to freedom and resurrection.

I did not have to search long or far for a healing venue. My neighbors Jonathan and Caroline, who lived on a back road in our village, ran a small retreat center from their home. They hosted teachers from various traditions, and although I had never attended a workshop at their center, I was always interested in the offerings they posted on-line. I admired and appreciated the work they did, the gift they offered to the greater community. I thought I remembered one of my colleagues talking about a healing circle she had attended led by Jonathan, and I decided to call her for details.

Before I made contact with my friend, however, I ran into Jonathan and Caroline on the road. They were heading home from a winter walk as I was starting out. I told them that I'd heard they hosted a healing group and that Neil and I were interested in exploring all options to healing what remained of his tumor. As we stood in the cold, they told me a bit about the healing practice that Jonathan conducted every Thursday evening in their living room for anyone who wanted to join them. It was called Tong Ren, and they were very enthusiastic about it. They would love to have Neil and me participate and were eager to help us in any way they could.

I felt that our meeting that day was serendipitous. I was seeking, and they appeared on the path before me. The convenience of their location, within walking distance of our home, was a major appeal. How much of a hardship would it be for Neil to walk down the road with me on a frosty evening, sit in a warm and welcoming space, and soak up the goodness of loving intentions?

The very next Thursday Neil and I were seated on Jonathan and Caroline's couch, in the company of five other participants who showed up either regularly or now and then to focus on their health or general well-being. Caroline told the group that earlier in the day she had received a phone call from Dorothy, a woman in our community with a degenerative disease. Although Dorothy could not venture out in this frigid weather, she wished to be included in the session. Neil and I were told that because Tong Ren is a form of energy therapy, drawing on Jung's theory of the "collective unconscious," it is often practiced to benefit even those who cannot be physically present at a session. Because the practice is believed to access energy from this universal source and direct it to the patient, and because no physical contact is involved or required, it is touted as an effective vehicle for distance healing.

Because we were new to the practice, Jonathan shared aspects of the routine he was about to begin. He told us that the founder of Tong Ren, who is a Boston-based, Chinese acupuncturist named Tom Tam, began working with a patient whose body, for some reason, was not able to accept the traditional needles that are inserted at key points to stimulate healing. Tam experimented with a small plastic anatomical model as an energetic representation of this patient. The doll-sized model, which I believe is used by students studying traditional acupuncture, is now available for practitioners like Jonathan to purchase. This small human form is labeled with letters and numbers which represent the meridians in our human bodies.

During his initial experimentation, Tom Tam inserted the needles in the same spot on the anatomical doll where he would have placed them in his client's body. He soon discovered that his human patient displayed the same healing benefits Tam would have expected had he inserted the needles internally. Eventually, Tam found it useful and effective to switch from the embedding of needles into the doll to tapping on each marked trigger point with a lightweight, magnetic hammer. I learned through doing a little research that the practice is based on the belief that disease is related to blockages in the body's essential flow of chi or life force. Tong Ren seeks to dissolve these block-ages, restoring the body's natural ability to heal itself, even when illnesses are chronic, debilitating, or incurable.

Jonathan had discovered Tong Ren while seeking relief from a health issue of his own. Although his problem was not life threatening, it compromised the quality of his life and became a priority for him to address. After his first session of Tong Ren, he noticed some improvement. He continued attending sessions and was so impressed with his progress and eventual healing that he decided to become trained in the practice in order to help others. He was enthusiastic about Tong Ren's compatibility with traditional healing modalities. Doing a combination of treatments, he assured us, was no problem.

As we sat, I quietly described to Neil the white, plastic, Barbie-sized model and the small hammer on the table in front of Jonathan. Also on the table was a huge manual with a list of every possible ailment. Each ailment listed is followed by a letter and number which corresponds to the numbers and letters stamped onto the model's body. Jonathan would use the model like a 3-D map, find the targeted trigger point on its body which corresponded to each of our conditions and begin tapping.

Neil and I sat side by side holding hands, something we often did in those days. We were engaging in an activity we had no experience with. I can't say that either of us was nervous or uncomfortable. But I think we had the feeling that we were in this together, that neither of us would have been there without the other. Our physical closeness seemed to seal that bond.

Jonathan, in his gentle and compassionate manner, addressed Patty. "Patty, how are you doing? What is challenging you right now? What would you like to focus on in your healing tonight?" Patty responded that she was experiencing tinnitus in both ears. It was an aggravating condition to live with. Sometimes the condition seemed to clear and it was a relief. Then it would return full force and wear her out. Jonathan consulted his manual, located the correct spot on the doll's head and began to tap. We sat quietly, just being present in the group. When Jonathan finished tapping for Patty's condition, he asked, "How are you feeling, Patty?" She responded, "I'm feeling relaxed and open." "I'm glad," said Jonathan.

And so it went, around the circle. Wendell was dealing with pain from arthritis. Sue was living with extreme nervousness about an ongoing, unpleasant issue at work. The emotional turmoil was starting to affect her on a physical level. Jonathan addressed the man sitting next to Neil. "Art, what's going on?" Art shared that he was feeling a bit run down this past week and could feel the whisper of a cold coming on. Jonathan began tapping.

It was Neil's turn. "Neil, tell us about yourself and why you are here tonight."

"Well, I have a malignant brain tumor—not as big as it used to be. But now I'm blind. And, oh yeah—I'm taking chemotherapy for a year."

Believe me, a lot of tapping followed Neil's introduction: one portion for the remaining tumor, one for the effects of chemo and radiation, and a third for the possible improvement of his eyesight.

I have learned in life that suffering is suffering. Each of our fellow human being's pain, hardship, or worry is deserving of respect and compassion. I do not stand in judgment of another's pain just I do not want my own to be judged or measured. It is all real. But so is the irreverent Taylor sense of humor. When we got home, Jim wanted to know how it went. Something in our retelling—maybe the juxtaposition of a sniffle with a tumor—made him burst out laughing. And it infected us. We caught his hilarity and experienced the deep release of a shared belly-laugh.

Despite our seeming irreverence, I felt strong and confident. Moving ahead with purpose, as we had at Jonathan and Caroline's, was a tonic for me. I believed it was possible that Neil's chi was beginning to shift, to move, to make space for his body to reclaim its wholeness.

~

In addition to our Thursday evenings at Tong Ren, Neil and I practiced some visualization together. Jessica's friend Amy had sent him a handful of healing stones in the mail. They were highly polished, of various colors and sizes, and each was taped to a card on which Amy had written its name and its healing properties.

One was an obvious "Neil" stone. It was larger than the others, a smooth, masculine brown with black streaks and specks, and most special, it was gently curved at an angle that fit perfectly against the side of his head. I felt drawn to this stone and wanted to use it. And so we started a ritual. Every night before we went to bed, we both kissed the stone. I then slid it gently back and forth across the scar that ran from the front of Neil's ear to the top of his head. As the stone slid over his skull, we visualized his tumor shrinking and disappearing. Our ritual took all of a minute or two, but it brought comfort to both of us. We were agents of healing because we were sent a stone meant for that purpose and because in our use of it we believed that healing was possible.

Visualization actually started for us in the earliest days at University-North—maybe even that first night in the emergency room when the intern from neurology viewed Neil's MRI. The description of his brain tumor being the size of a small orange was pronounced then or in the days immediately following. I can't pinpoint the "who said" or the "where we were," but the image of an orange was born and took shape. For Neil, it seemed to give the situation a reality. The evil abstract now had a form. He could picture it. And those close to us could too. Neil was harboring a tumor the size of an orange.

When Dr.Carrington, his surgeon, met with us immediately following the operation and told us that he had removed about seventy percent of the tumor, the remaining thirty to be treated with chemo and radiation, I told Neil, when he was finally conscious again, that the tumor had been reduced to about the size of a walnut. It felt better than an orange. Months later, when a friend from college called to check on him, the first thing Neil heard was, "Buddy—such great news—I hear your tumor is the size of a blueberry!" I exploded with laughter when Neil told me. Yes, his progress was going well; his tumor was responding to treatment and shrinking—but a blueberry? Who in our wide network coined that one and passed it along? I loved it—could picture that tiny thing. Yay, fruit! The smaller you get, the sweeter you are.

MY FAMILY PUT A HUGE EFFORT into keeping me busy during the time I spent alone. It was essential to them that each day I had an activity to engage in or a goal to strive for, something to keep my mind and body busy as a remedy to keep me from falling into depression. There was no way my mother could be at peace leaving me alone for the entire day while she and my father were at work if she thought I was lonely, miserable, and hopeless about my future.

The fact that Mom taught at a small elementary school just down the road from our house turned out to be a godsend for both of us. There was nowhere I felt more comfortable than in a classroom full of children. In addition to my experience at Greenwood, I had been a seasoned substitute teacher at the public school I had attended in my youth. Both my mother, who taught first and second grades, and her teaching partners Dena and Marjorie, who had third and fourth graders, were happy to have me volunteer and were eager for their students to know me—someone with a huge challenge who was facing life head on. Volunteering in these two classrooms during a potentially lonely year for me provided the opportunity to interact with others, big and little alike. It also gave me a great opportunity to practice my mobility skills with my cane as I walked down the road from my house to the school. I was a rank beginner back then, but it was literally a straight shot, three hundred yards down a paved rural road where my mom would be watching and waiting at the door to greet me. The kids were always excited to see me and were full of curiosity, asking me every question imaginable about being blind—"How long have you been blind, what is the cane for, can you see anything at all?"—unlike most adults who probably have similar questions but are too shy or sensitive to ask. I found it all so refreshing and fun. The kids were open and innocent, still free from making judgments about my limitations due to my unusual and "interesting" disability.

In both classrooms I was set up to work with small groups of some of the strongest readers. My job was to assess and stretch their comprehension. As they took turns reading and then discussing what they'd read, nudged by questions from me, I couldn't help but be impressed by them. I, too, had been a strong, early reader, but it felt to me as if they had me beat! Those mornings, of course, brought me back to my days of working with my Greenwood boys, and it seemed so long ago though, in truth, it wasn't. My gratitude goes out to my young friends at the Westminster West School for giving me the chance to practice again, even for a couple of hours a week. I think back to our massive group hugs when it was time for me to head home, promising that I'd return the following week. I can still feel the warmth.

~

My mother hates it when I sometimes refer to my scheduled activities during the full year of my treatment as "killing time," and she almost always corrects me. It wasn't killing time, it was filling time. And, really, she is right.

My comings and goings, my learning new things, my giving and my receiving all involved some degree of social contact. However, there was one major piece that was solitary by nature, involved just me, myself and I, and was hugely important to my future competence in my new life. That activity was learning to type. If I was to be at all successful using the JAWS program specifically designed for the blind population, I simply had to be able to type easily, quickly, and competently. And this activity, which filled or killed lots of time in the solitude of my parents' home, was one that I really enjoyed.

My father ordered a decent typing tutor program and set it up on our home computer. Having hours on my hands to use my always vivid imagination, I conjured dreams of becoming the most proficient person ever behind a keyboard. I remembered how secretaries used to brag about how many words they could type in a minute, and I was revved up to double that number, whatever it was. In my standard fashion I devoted almost every waking hour when I was alone to mastering this skill. If you're wondering about my past as a high school student, college student, and teacher, I have a small confession to make. I'd never learned to type until I was forced to by becoming blind. I spent my four years of college typing fifteen page papers using the old hunt and peck technique with my two index fingers. I had to stop every half hour or so to give those working fingers a rest before they cramped up on me.

I learned from my new program that the F and the J buttons have a little tactile dot or bar on them. This goes for every computer in existence. Most people never notice this and are skeptical when you tell them. Go ahead—I'll give you a minute to check your own computer—pretty cool, right? I like to think this little detail was designed so that blind people can orient themselves to any keyboard—either that or so sighted people can type in the dark. In any case, my typing tutor program started me with just a few keys. After I became proficient typing "nab a cab" or "a bad lad gabs," I graduated to twisters like "Jolly jester Jerry Johnson juggled a jiggling jug of juice in the Jamaican jungle and jeered at a jovial jaguar." OK—that might be a bit of an exaggeration, but you get the idea. It took a sizable chunk of time to complete the program, and when I was done I don't think I could have broken any speed records, but I could type proficiently and that was the whole point.

*a*THROUGHOUT NEIL'S YEAR OF HEALING, friends and family marveled at how well he was managing. He was able to stick to his calendar of activities without interruption. He never missed social engagements. He became connected to life via his auditory sense, through National Public Radio and his growing competency with adaptive technology. His speaking computer, his Victor Stream Reader which held downloaded copies of fiction and non-fiction, his phone—these were his lifelines.

Neil had never been a particularly "tech-y" type guy, so becoming familiar and becoming comfortable navigating the parts of this world that were new to him presented a steep learning curve. He experienced times of extreme frustration and times of great satisfaction in his growing competency with the technological advances that were available to the blind community.

In addition, there were other adjustments Neil had to contend with that first year, ones that required him to make shifts in his very nature. The first was that despite our greatest efforts to construct an active life, Neil did, in the end, spend much time alone. Jim and I would go off to our jobs and be gone for most of the day. Each day one of his instructors would arrive for a session, or his driver, Robyn, would arrive to transport him to a massage session or therapy appointment. On the way home they'd stop for errands or lunch. But these appointments and outings did not fill a day and could not make up for the busyness and collaboration that comprise a regular work day, the kind that Neil had had just months before.

The second major adjustment was that Neil was forced to practice patience, an attribute that was not natural to his quicksilver temperament and the nervous system he was born with. A life of blindness requires coming to terms with the fact that you must exist differently in the world than almost anyone else. Your lot is to wait for others to pick you up for an outing, develop the gentlest touch in reaching for something so as not to spill or break it, train your body to move mindfully in an effort to keep safe, ask for help when you've misplaced something, be accompanied by another to purchase food in a supermarket. My admiration for Neil is huge and my compassion even greater when I recognize that he had to make conscious decisions every day about monitoring his inner frustrations and resentments so as not to alienate those around him. Neil was born with a good measure of sunshine and optimism, but how many times, I wonder, did he and does he, play-act cheerfulness when he is feeling just the opposite?

SEVEN

BEGIN AGAIN

Though your destination is not clear
Unfurl yourself into the grace of beginning

~ John O' Donohue

EACH ENDEAVOR THAT FIRST YEAR HAD an element of trial and error attached to it. In our family's joint efforts to construct a satisfying life for Neil we struggled to re-figure activities that had been important to him, that had defined who he was. Was it possible for him to reclaim any part of his past, or would he have to rethink it all and start again, a new and different Neil? These were the questions that confronted us each day.

The conversation Neil and I had had just prior to his surgery haunted me. I remembered the fear in his eyes as he contemplated the possibility of never riding his mountain bike again. At the time I was able to soften his "what if" question with its unlikelihood. I couldn't think of anything that would stand in the way of his passion other than the temporary treatment for his tumor. But what were the possibilities now? Could he ever ride again? Could he still ski? Could he kayak or water ski? These questions became mini research projects during the year following Neil's release from the hospital.

*n*THE WINTER OF MY YEAR OF HEALING, while I was living with my parents and undergoing treatment, I got a call from the father of one of my former Greenwood students. He was calling to tell me that he'd just been certified to guide blind skiers by outfitting them with earphones through which he could call out directions as they skied together. He was eager to gain experience in his new training and wanted to know if I'd like to try it.

Having grown up in Vermont, I'd started skiing at the age of six. The year after graduating from college I'd spent the winter working and skiing in Alta, Utah. Skiing was in my blood. In Utah, I'd loved skiing in the glades and woods, routinely jumping off cliffs and even mastering back flips in the powder that blankets the mountains of western ski areas. Of course I knew that now, in my sorry state, everything was different. But the memories of those days enticed me, and I was willing to put all that fancy stuff aside just to get out on the slopes and try to ski again. So I said yes to the Greenwood dad.

My mother drove me to Mount Snow where he was waiting. He handed me a pinny to wear that identified me as a blind skier. As I pulled it over my parka, my dignity, my sense of myself, was bruised a bit, but hey—I was out here to ski, and if this is what it took, then so be it. As he hooked me up with the earphones, he described the speaker that would connect us. And it really hit me. I'd be skiing using my auditory sense instead of my visual.

The long and short of it is that it was way more difficult than I could have imagined. I'd always taken my coordination for granted, had been a natural athlete, but now, on this first day skiing blind, everything seemed purely mechanical. I was reduced to relying solely on a voice with commands—"left, right, left, more left."

We started out going down easy little groomers where, just like I remember in my sighted days, the snowboarders were sitting on the trail. But now I had to weave around them without being able to see them. My balance was still terrible, and without working eyes I had no way of judging the pitch of the slope. I would lean too far into my turns and consequently take these crunching falls on my hips—really painful falls. I tried to act like they didn't hurt. The first few times I'd say, "Hey—no problem. I'm OK." But it kept happening consistently, and I thought to myself, "Why the hell am I doing this?" The experience became excruciating, physically, mentally, and emotionally.

I took two more rides on the chairlift, even though my heart wasn't in it anymore. I did it because my guide, who was such a sincere and nice guy, had paid for my ticket and I felt obliged to give it my best shot. But I decided on one of those chairlift rides that I would never do this again. Skiing was done for me. I'd loved it so much, but now, fumbling along in such an altered way just made me nostalgic for what had been. What I had left from my skiing days were good and happy memories, and this day was ruining all of that.

Mom, of course, felt badly about how the day played out. She feared that her initial enthusiasm for the venture had pushed me into something I wasn't ready for, that the state of my body, under the influence of chemotherapy, and my inexperience with navigating any environment as a blind person had doomed me to failure. How had we fallen victim to naivete and unrealistic expectations?

But I told her no. I had discovered that I would never be able to ski the way I used to ski and, in this case, I couldn't compromise. The adjustment brought me no pleasure, no gratification. Yes, it was sad, but it was just one more sadness in the ever-expanding line-up displayed front and center in my new life.

*a*SINCE NEIL'S DISAPPOINTING EXPERIENCE ON the slopes I've learned a bit more about blind athletes. It seems that most who successfully plow down mountains on skis or do other extreme sports have been blind from birth or from a young age. The world they inhabit is the world they have known always. A twenty-eight year old who becomes blind overnight finds himself in a dark, frightening, unpredictable world without benefit of his other senses having had a chance to move to the forefront. Everything requires practice, even the simplest things. Nothing can be taken for granted, and the living of daily life is exhausting.

The first time we cross-country skied ended pretty much like the downhill day. One Saturday I convinced a reluctant Neil to accompany me to a touring center near our home where

I'd skied for many years with the kids in my elementary school. We started out on the easiest route—flat land and two very gentle hills groomed the "classical" way, with two side-by-side tracks like a ready made pathway designed to hold your skis in position. Of course, I didn't know what I was doing, but I had good instincts and how hard could it be? My thought was that Neil would really like the feel of his skis being guided by the grooves. They would give him support—a tactile aid.

But ski tracks are never perfect. One can kind of fade out and lose its clear edge. Then your foot slides away from the other one in an uncoordinated manner, compromising your balance. And that kept happening to Neil. Without vision, he could not just look down and step back into the track. What I thought and hoped would act as a frame of reference was too unreliable. The track was just plain frustrating.

We climbed the first gentle hill, turned around, and faced downward. Here there was no track, and I felt relieved to be free of it. Several days after this first outing I read that a successful way to accompany a blind skier down an open slope is to extend a ski pole horizontally in front of both of you, take hold of it together, and descend as one. But I hadn't read that yet. So I said, "OK, Neil, this is pretty gentle. Go ahead." He shoved off, but instead of heading straight, he veered off to the side which was icy, lost his balance from the changed texture of the snow, and crashed down on the back of his head. So now he pretty much hated everything about the experience, and we shortly headed home.

But I wasn't going to give up on this yet. I felt as though I had learned a lot from the outing—mostly what not to do—and I knew I could avoid or improve on some of my mistakes. In the days that followed, we got a couple of inches of fresh, light, fluffy snow and the conditions were perfect. I convinced Neil to try again on the open field down the road from our house. I borrowed two elastic bracelets of large jingle bells from the music room of my school and pulled one onto each of my arms so that Neil could hear me without always having to talk. And then I said, "There's nothing you can run into here—there's also no trail, no track, just soft snow. Know that if you come close to hitting something I'll tell you—but there isn't anything. Now go."

And he did. And I stopped him when we came to even a slight incline, just to tell him the lay of the land ahead. And our cheeks got red and we laughed and he actually said he was having fun. Yes! Success!

n WITHOUT A DOUBT, THE SADDEST PASSION torn from my life was down-hill biking. It never mattered to me that my friends weren't into it. I would make solo trips to Mount Snow and ride the chairlift over and over enjoying the spectacular scenery of summertime Vermont. Being by myself actually made the experience more intense. I would barrel down that mountain, overjoyed by the stimulation, reveling in the high that comes with brushing up against a bit of danger. After losing my sight, I knew I could never hope to do that again, just racing against myself down a steep mountain trail. But I could try tandem biking.

I had a good friend, Rich, about a generation older than me, who became one of my supports during my year in Westminster West, and he was an avid rider. He owned a tandem bike and was excited to take me out riding. On that first trip, how could I not compare the experience to the downhill riding I had loved so much? It didn't bring me that powerful adrenaline rush, but I had to admit that I did enjoy our outing together. Just to be sitting on a bike and pedaling, feeling the wind pushing against my body, feeling speed again, brought back some of what I used to feel.

During this intensive trial and error period of my life, Brad Ludden, the founder of an organization called First Descents, invited me to go on a five-borough, New York City bike ride. It was a fifty-two mile ride and he wanted us to do it together on a tandem bike. Unfortunately for me, thirty-two thousand other people participated in this fund-raising bike ride as well. The result of all this enthusiasm was that the whole event turned into a huge bike traffic jam and, consequently, a seemingly never-ending nightmare for me. We would go about a thousand yards, then have to stop our bike and wait for the traffic jam to start flowing again. So the whole trip consisted of stopping and starting, stopping and starting, which on a tandem is challenging because you have to start at exactly the same time, and it's a real balancing feat just to have successful starts. In addition, every time we had to stop and drop our feet to the ground the bike pedals would crash into my shins. They were taking a real beating. And my butt began to hurt due to proceeding like this for so many hours. So this was less of an athletic adventure and more of a monotony with pain included. Hardest of all, I couldn't people watch, which undoubtedly was a huge and engaging aspect of that day. I'm sure it was a grand visual experience, but I had none of that fun. I was just in darkness, starting and stopping, starting and stopping. It was a total buzz-kill.

~

Although I had become detached from many of the physical endeavors that once gave me pleasure and a sense of identity, I still could work out. Being blind had no effect on my ability to continue lifting. In addition, and a happy complement to lifting, I developed a new passion the year I lived with my parents: running on my father's elliptical running machine. Once upon a time I couldn't understand people who exercised on elliptical runners—like what was the point? It became that year, and remains, my main source of exercise. I put on some music, jump on my own elliptical now, and run for an hour, totally transported and "lost" in the music. I sweat profusely and breathe hard and my outlook on life shifts. Afterward, I feel like a new man. My day has just become brighter. I am uplifted.

EVERY PURSUIT WAS NEW, BECAUSE NEIL, in large part, was "new." And this new reality gave birth to a mental shift. I began to understand that while it's impossible not to mourn what is gone (Neil and I cried and cried the day of the annual neighborhood baseball game, an event which had made him a legend after he'd hit a home run that smacked the fire house across the street) it is possible to be thankful for what you have left, to accept less, and to view it with gratitude.

Slowly, Neil moved into that place. He began to appreciate the smaller pleasures: running with abandon on an empty beach; simple walks, hand-in-hand, down a Vermont country road; snow-shoeing, which replaced his once beloved skiing; and the king of all physical experiences now—his workout practice. Neil's commitment to this totally accessible form of exercise is astounding, as are the benefits. His body has become, once again, strong and athletic, and his outlook on life more optimistic. He is a classic survivor who has learned and embraces what works for him. Nothing keeps him from missing a day of exertion, of personal challenge, and the ultimate rewards they bring.

EIGHT

A CAST ASSEMBLES

Never forget that everyone needs encouragement.
And everyone who receives it—young or old,
successful or less-than-successful, unknown or famous—
is changed by it.

~ John C. Maxwell

a IN ADDITION TO NEIL'S THERAPIST, his massage contacts, Chloe and Ben, and Joe from Vermont Division for the Blind, an interesting array of players began to enter Neil's life. Some were on stage for a brief period and gone before we really knew them; others became part of the fabric of those days and will be remembered for their part in orienting Neil to a new reality.

Irving showed up first, sent by Joe to teach preliminary life skills that would help Neil gain some independence. He arrived with his driver due to his own visual impairment, and I could tell almost immediately that he was a man who loved his job. Irving's first order of business was to introduce Neil to several items that he thought would prove useful. Some of these aids did became helpful additions to Neil's life and others not so much.

The most helpful to our family in our respective roles of being the blind person and living with the blind person were sheets of spongy raised tactile dots with adhesive backs. Irving explained that they were tremendously helpful in enabling the blind to safely and independently operate household appliances. On our electric stove, for instance, we could adhere a raised dot to indicate where high heat was located. Neil could touch the dot with one hand, then turn the dial and line it up with the dot. We could adhere two dots to signify where "low" was located.

It would be melodramatic to say that the tactile dots opened up the world for Neil, but they did allow him to become more competent in the world inside our home. We became dot crazy. We fastened the dots on our washing machine, our thermostat, Neil's boom box, his tape recorder. Jessica and I loved finding new uses for the dots, and Neil enjoyed mastering whatever dot challenges we cooked up.

The second item Irving presented to Neil was a tiny box with prongs attached to one side. The tiny box held a battery. Irving and Neil were standing at the kitchen counter, and Irving asked me to get him a drinking glass and a pitcher of water. I watched him attach the prongs to the inside rim of the glass.

"OK, Neil, start pouring the water. Don't worry about spilling it. I'll let you know when to stop."

Neil began pouring. And Irving didn't need to stop him. As soon as the liquid reached the prongs, a god awful alarm went off. Neil stopped and I plugged my ears. Irving seemed delighted with the simplicity and effectiveness of the device. We thought it was the silliest invention in the world. Why would a thirsty blind person who wanted a glass of juice go fishing in a drawer for an alarm when he could simply place a finger inside the glass to feel when to stop pouring? The only time Neil used it was to show it to Jim that very night. Then we stuck it in a drawer where from time to time it would start squawking with no provocation. It did it one too many times, and we threw it out.

An aid that I thought was cool was an 8x10 template of thick cardboard that looked like a Venetian blind in that it had about ten long spaces cut out from top to bottom. It was to be placed over a sheet of paper and used as a tactile aid to keep a blind person's handwriting from zig-zagging all over the place. What it couldn't do, however, was help the writer judge the spacing between words. In truth, the aid was a bit anti-quated. Computers have been a boon and a blessing to the blind community, replacing not all but many of the aids which served in the past. Neil could do all of his writing on the computer. The only time I thought the template might be handy was in writing a birthday or wedding card to a friend. But somehow we never had it when we needed it, it was a bit too large to fit a greeting card format, and Neil preferred just having someone put his finger in a good starting place. His sentences definitely took the shape of hills and valleys, but he didn't care.

*O*THER THINGS IRVING SHOWED ME WERE much more useful. On his second visit, he demonstrated how to fold money in order to distinguish the denomination of each bill. In the United States, paper currency is a real challenge for the blind in that all our bills feel identical to each other. In Australia and Malaysia, each denomination has a distinct width and length. In Canada, paper currency now sports braille dots in one corner so that blind Canadians can quickly "read" the denominations of each bill they are giving and receiving. Because neither of these helpful aids have been adopted in the United States, the blind community has had to devise its own system. One dollar bills are left unfolded in the wallet; five dollar bills are folded in half lengthwise; ten dollar bills are folded in half by width; twenty dollar bills in half by length and again in half by width. This method, of course, is completely dependent on a sighted person first identifying the denomination the blind person is about to fold, but it's the best we have to date. I didn't even want to ask about receiving change.

It was all pretty interesting, and I adhered to the practice at first. Then I found it too time consuming to commit to. Now I just arrange my money stacked according to its value. And most of the time I simply use my credit card.

Back in the kitchen, Irving was impressed to see that we had already decorated the dials with the raised tactile dots he'd given us earlier. He was ready to teach me the safety precautions that blind cooks should never short cut. First off, a burner should never be turned on until the pot is carefully positioned on the burner, stirring spoon in place within it. Secondly, the pot handle should never be facing out as it could inadvertently be bumped, causing an accident involving boiling water on unsuspecting skin or a pot of potentially lethal pasta crashing to the floor. During the whole lesson I punctuated Irving's presentation with pertinent, well thought out questions. When we were through I excused myself to use the bathroom. While making my way back to the kitchen to rejoin him and his driver and my mother, I congratulated myself on how smoothly I was starting to navigate my childhood home. I was really beginning to get this blind thing down. Always the student wanting to please, I hoped Irving noticed.

I entered the kitchen and successfully located the chair I'd been sitting in. I put my hand on the arm rest while quickly picking up the thread of conversation they were engaged in. And then, CRASH! My body hit the floor and landed on top of a large plastic bag filled with recyclables ready to be taken to the shed beyond the kitchen. The sound of my unexpected landing brought the conversation to an abrupt halt as my mother and the driver ran to my side to help me up. Everyone asked me again and again if I was all right. I quickly laughed, making a dumb joke, trying to divert the embarrassing attention from myself.

"Yes, I'm fine, really— thank you."

They set me back in the chair I'd intended to sit in, and Irving's voice, kind and supportive, cut through the ringing in my ears.

"Neil—it's OK. These things happen. Please don't be hard on yourself."

I had made the ultimate misjudgment I'd been warned about soon after losing my sight. While basking in my confidence and congratulating myself on my growing sense of orientation, I thought I had placed my hand on the right arm rest—picture me facing the chair—which would have centered me to the seat as I pivoted around. But, instead, I had unsuspectingly and carelessly grabbed the left one. Consequently, I sat where there was no seat—nothing to catch my butt but the floor.

The truth, of course, was that I was far from all right. The confidence I had felt just a few minutes earlier was instantly sucked out of me. It was as though I had been sailing courageously at top speed in my new ship when suddenly the strong wind died, causing my proud, billowing sail to completely deflate. I was left, miserable and shriveled, and I could smell the stale aroma of beer from the recycling, now emanating from the backside on my wet shorts. If I had thought, even for a moment, that I was making my peace with or making my way with this whole blindness package, it was blatantly clear that I was totally wrong.

I recall standing up briefly, shaking hands with Irving and his driver and sitting back down on the godforsaken chair while my mom showed them to the door. When she returned to the kitchen, I was already getting choked up by the humiliation of the whole ordeal. Mom reached for me, saying that everything was going to be OK, that we were in this together and would be, every step of the way. I nodded, weakly, as my grief overtook me, and I began to sob. Nothing was OK, and it never would be. My mother put her arms around me, and I could feel her tears on my own wet cheek. As always, my sorrow was her sorrow, my pain was hers, and we rocked back and forth together. This seemingly small mishap had brought everything to a head. Everything that had once been second nature to me now took an almost insurmountable effort to achieve, and when things fell apart—plain failed—like they had today, it was just too hard to handle. And I couldn't help but feel in those painful moments following Irving's departure, without words passing between us, that my mother was holding her once tough, independent, twenty-nine year old son that tightly so as not to let what remained of him slip away.

We wept together for a long time, our chests rising and falling in a rhythm of despair until we had no more tears to cry. After releasing the emotions that I had hidden behind a false stoicism, I felt a great relief, as if the discharge of all those tears had cleansed me from the toxicity of holding and hiding such immense sorrow. This was a pivotal moment in my life. I knew I wouldn't and couldn't ever again pretend that what I had gone through had not taken a huge toll on me. I had no shame for crying into my mother's arms. I understood, on the heels of that kitchen drama, that taking care of myself meant more than tending and healing my body. Taking care of myself emotionally and spiritually held equal weight.

AFTER HIS SECOND SESSION WITH NEIL, Joe called to tell us that Irving had been offered a job in northern Vermont. He would continue working with the blind and visually impaired, but the position being offered up north appealed to him and he was moving on. Neil and I agreed that we wished him well, and, at the same time, Neil expressed some relief about taking a break from life skills. Irving had been a compassionate presence, especially after Neil's humiliating fall, but there was something about Irving's fervor that he was not ready for. Neil was still reeling from the events of his life, those that had occurred so recently and those he was preparing to face in the near future. His inner reserves had limits, and we needed to recognize and respect them. So when Joe suggested that Maxine, Neil's braille teacher, take over life skills, Neil said no. He would practice what he had learned from Irving with his family, at least for the time being. I thought about Joe's cautionary advise when Neil first arrived home. Perhaps he was right; taking on too much too soon was not wise.

~

Maxine began coming to the house to teach Neil the foundations of braille. Learning braille at the age of twenty-nine, in the year 2008, when technological advances were happening almost daily, wasn't really that essential. Neil would never read a book in braille. That would take years of study given that the language has many abbreviations and shortcuts besides the twenty-six raised dot letters. The audio world of today is huge and accessible and used by the blind and sighted alike. Likewise, typing on a computer outfitted with the program JAWS, widely used by the blind community, enables the blind to listen to the text they write, eliminating the necessity of typing on a braille typewriter. We were told that Neil would be learning "functional" braille, enough to aid him in practical areas of his life. He might want to label his food shelves, clothing drawers or medicine bottles. Maxine supplied him with a hand-held label maker, the end product being a tape with a sticky back and raised braille dots.

For several months, Neil became obsessed with braille. It was a language, a code to crack, and it seemed to take the place of his former love of word scrambles and scrabble. He was intrigued with the way a simple grid of six circles arranged in two parallel lines of three circles each (think of dice) became a letter based on which of the circles were highlighted. And "highlighted" for the blind, of course, is based on touch, the tactile sense. The particular arrangements of raised dots within the grid became Neil's new ABCs.

Neil roped me into learning the braille alphabet with him. Games are no fun unless you have a partner, and saying "I don't feel like it" to Neil was not possible for me. So we learned together. Maxine had given Neil a set of small plastic braille alphabet tiles, and they became our favorite learning tool. We tested each other constantly. Neil would hand me a tile, and with my eyes closed I would feel for the number and placement of the raised dots. The beginning letters of the alphabet were fairly easy to memorize; the letters toward the end of the alphabet used more dots in more complicated patterns and were more challenging. The flip side of our "reading" the letters with our fingers was testing each other on the formation of each letter as if we were attempting to write in braille by searching for the letter on a braille typewriter. Neil would say, "R..," and I would answer, "one, two, three, five," naming the circles that would be raised in order to represent the letter R. And we did practice on the braille typewriter. We would take turns typing words or very short sentences and try to decipher them back to each other. As we reminisced recently about those days of playing with the alphabet tiles, Neil told me that they marked the beginning of his moving his tactile sense to the forefront of how he needed to operate in the world.

Maxine, herself, was by no means a braille expert. It didn't take Neil long to realize, or at least to feel, that she was only a few steps ahead of him. That may have been the case, but Maxine had the curriculum guide, and she provided the structure of the weekly lessons. She gave Neil a giant white Braille "primer" in which he was supposed to practice between lessons. The primer introduced three or four letters over several lessons, then combined them to form simple words: at, cat, act, as, scat, cast. Eventually enough letters were introduced to enable sentences to be presented. And that's where I fell down. Concentrating as hard as possible I could not reliably feel where one letter ended and the next started. The discrete letters I had memorized so diligently on the individual plastic squares—those simple and complex array of dots—seemed to melt into the neighboring dots of the next letter. It wasn't hard to feel the spaces between words, but the spaces between letters within a word were beyond my oafish tactile sensibilities. Neil was better, but not a lot. I felt somewhat better when I learned that the primers in Neil's possession were not new. They had been handed down from other Braille learners, and Maxine told us that braille books eventually get somewhat worn down. It makes sense, but whoever would have imagined that fact as an issue in blind education?

In the end, Neil learned enough under Maxine's tutelage so that when he eventually entered The Carroll Center for the Blind for a four month study of independent living skills, he tested higher in his knowledge of braille than most of the other students. He went to the top of the class. We laughed. His hard work and my side-kick supporting role paid off!

I look at those days of Neil becoming familiar with braille from a multidimensional perspective. Although he never uses it now in any area of his life, it served some important purposes back then. First, it gave him something to do at a time when most activities in his life were lost to him. Second, practicing with the raised-dot tiles helped develop his tactile sense. And, third, it was a great brain game for him, requiring lots of work with symbols, pattern and memory.

One winter day during our year as housemates, Neil and I were sitting in the kitchen about an hour before Jim was due home from work. Neil had been out earlier in the day with his friend Em. They'd had lunch in downtown Brattleboro and decided to do a little shopping at Sam's Outdoor Outfitters before heading home. Neil had been a guy who had always liked clothes, a guy who had the interest, patience, and temperament to go on shopping expeditions with his girl friend or me back in the day. But who wouldn't expect all that to have changed after he lost his ability to see? When he became blind and was taking his first tentative steps toward independent living, we were told that many blind people decide to stick to one color for most of their shirts and purchase all black or all brown pants to avoid confusion and embarrassing color combinations. But that could never be Neil. He has remained a clothes horse through thick and through thin. It still gives him pleasure and a sense of identity.

As he pulled a pair of forest-green Dickie trousers out of his shopping bag that afternoon, I said, "Neil, you already have two pairs of Dickies you bought last month."

He answered, "True, but I didn't have a green pair, so now I have a blue pair, a black pair and a green pair."

"Great," I shot back, "and how do you propose to tell them apart when you get dressed in the morning?"

"I don't know," he admitted, though he didn't seem too concerned about it.

All of a sudden and out of nowhere, but perhaps born of the fact that I was becoming more and more creative in dealing with daily challenges, an idea, a possible solution to the clothing ID dilemma washed over me, and I became very excited.

"Neil," I gasped, "I have an idea. Sit tight—actually, no! Get me those two other pairs of pants."

While he did my bidding, I ran to get my sewing basket. I felt like a scientist ready to test my theory, my brainchild, confident of my brilliance and eager to share my results with the general public. What my nimble mind was working on was a way to use braille to help Neil identify his clothing. I remembered that in the early seventies crewel work, a fancy type of embroidery with a wide array of creative stitches, was very popular in the craft world. I had made several crewel-work pillows during that period and had even embroidered hippy-type peasant blouses for myself and work shirts for Jim. And one of those stitches—one of the simplest to learn and the only one I still remembered by heart after more than thirty years—was the French knot, a nubby RAISED dot.

Rifling through my sewing basket, I found some left over embroidery floss. I threaded a length of green floss into the thickest needle I had and poked it into the inside waistband of Neil's green trousers. I twisted the floss deftly around the needle two times, plunged it back through the cloth, and formed a perfect French knot. I touched it with my thumb. It stood tall and proud—a cloth version of a braille dot.

My motivation soared. I said, "Neil, tell me the braille formation of the letter G!"

He said, "One, two, four, five."

I retorted, "Yup, and one, two, four, five forms a perfect little square. I'm sewing the letter G into the waistband of your green pants, and when I'm done I want you to feel the cloth dots and tell me if you recognize the G."

I handed him the finished product, showed him where to touch and he let out a joyful whoop.

"I can't believe it! That's so awesome! How did you do that? How did you know how?"

We were both thrilled. I was on a roll, powered by a creative high. We decided that we would use the letter B for the color blue and BK for black. Into the waistband of the black pants I formed the dots one and two (picture the first two vertical dots on the game die); then I left a space and formed the K (dots one and three, vertically). I handed Neil the pants, and he said, "Clear as day—B and K, black." When I finished sewing the blue pair, I tested him several times, randomly handing him green pants, blue pants, black pants. He scored with one hundred percent accuracy.

Five minutes later Jim walked in the door. I said casually, "Hey look, Neil has three different colors of the same brand of pants. He's developed a sixth sense. He'll tell you which color is which. I don't know how he does it."

Neil hammed it up, gave a marvelous performance, and Jim was flabbergasted. "How does he do that? What's going on? Tell me!"

Neil and I hooted and hollered like exclusive friends with a private joke. Finally we showed Jim the French knots, and, once again, I got to revel in accolades of my cleverness, my ingenuity. I couldn't conjure even a shred of modesty or humility, so, what the heck, I grinned from ear to ear. That was a good day.

~

Undoubtedly, the most essential skill for Neil to begin learning following his release from Southside Rehabilitation Center was mobility. The loss of being able to make one's way in the world, to move with ease from place to place, to feel physically safe in space is staggering. Not only are the newly blind stripped of the dearest of the five senses, they are stripped of their freedom.

Within a week of Neil's return home, Joe Stein sent Cliff Shears, an experienced mobility trainer, to meet Neil and to give us advice on ways to adapt the physical layout of our house to accommodate him. Cliff appeared at our door on the appointed day, tall, gangly, and loose-jointed, but graceful at the same time. He wore an ever-present baseball cap over his red hair. He seemed to have an easy way about him, was someone who felt comfortable in anyone's kitchen, confident in what he did and who he was.

From my perspective, Cliff taught us a lot that very first day. He reiterated how fortunate it was that Neil was returning to a house he had lived in for years and urged Neil to see, in his mind's eye, the layout he had once taken for granted, a layout he knew intimately but had never had to "picture" before his blindness. He told us that the blind generally do not "cane" in their homes. They internalize the layout and just walk, using their hands outstretched for protection in open spaces and the walls to guide them on familiar routes, from kitchen to bathroom to bedroom. He once again demonstrated "sighted guide" for me, and I had an "ah-ha" moment as I saw that I was being too stiff and self-conscious in the way I guided Neil with my arm bent close to my own body as if it was up to me to be completely in charge. Cliff demonstrated that a guide does nothing more than keep his or her arm in a straight-down, relaxed position, the way it would hang naturally if you were walking alone. The blind person lightly holds the guide's upper arm. When the three of us ventured upstairs, Cliff showed us how to walk through a door or through a tight space by relaying a non-verbal signal.

He simply moved his arm to the small of his back, palm up, and Neil got the message to walk behind Cliff rather than at his side.

Mobility training with Cliff was added to Neil's calendar at once and took on great importance for all of us. Jessica and I, in particular, wanted to learn as much as we could in order to help Neil with this immense challenge. Cliff and Neil worked inside our home, in our neighborhood, and in the gymnasium of a local elementary school where Neil could practice maintaining a straight line while walking a fairly long distance, a skill that was difficult for him.

*n*AMONG MY REHABILITATION TEAM WAS Cliff Shears whose formidable job it was to teach me how to get around with a cane. At first his robust masculinity suited me just fine. He reminded me of lacrosse coaches I'd had in the past—guys with an upbeat, easy, "can-do" demeanor. I promised myself that I would work just as hard as a mobility student as I had years ago at the try-outs for the University of Vermont lacrosse team as an unknown walk-on. I would show the same tenaciousness and perseverance that had earned me a spot on the team.

After Cliff's introduction and breakdown of what we were going to cover in our lessons together and what he expected of me as his student, I was inspired by his no-nonsense vigor to teach, and I appreciated what, at first, I thought was a sardonic sense of humor. But after a number of sessions, Cliff started to make me feel unsettled. Initially, I second-guessed my feelings, attributed them to my vulnerability and rawness in the face of the traumatic turn my life had taken. I shrugged off his seemingly thoughtless remarks, even attributing my over-sensitivity to my recent brain surgery and radiation treatment. But, somehow, my mind would always go back to the fact that Cliff was the professional who was charged not only with teaching me to become a proficient blind traveler but also with assuring me, through his vote of confidence, that my fledgling abilities would grow and improve. I probably wasn't his first client who had lost his sight suddenly and unexpectedly

During one of our first meetings I asked Cliff what it had been like training to be a mobility instructor for the blind. I asked whether the trainers were ever blindfolded to simulate the perspective of their clients. He quickly confirmed that, yes, they had been. And with seeming glee, he went on to describe how as soon as the clock struck three, he threw his blindfold to the wind, cast aside his cumbersome cane, and peeled out of the parking lot on his motorcycle, free at last. I felt acid rise to my throat. How was this description supposed to make a freshly blinded young man like me feel? Unlucky, from stem to stern? Wishing that I, too, could do the same? Was he so obtuse that he was incapable of "getting" how his jocularity in this retelling could bring on depression in me?

One day, at the end of a tiring session, Cliff asked me what kind of physical endeavors I was still interested in. It took me several moments to come up with an answer because so many of the things I had loved were now gone from my life. But I came up with one response, an activity that in my former life would only make me yawn. I answered, "hiking," thinking it was something I still could do or at least aspire to. The moment it left my mouth Cliff informed me, with much authority, that blind people are not really successful at hiking what with all the exposed tree roots and loose rocks underfoot on your average hiking trail. I was stunned into momentary silence. His proclamation felt like a hot slap across the face. But I rallied and informed him that I was currently listening to a book on tape, a memoir of a blind man who'd hiked the entire Appalachian Trail with only his guide dog as a companion. About as quickly as I'd interrupted him, he did the same to me, referring to the author of the memoir as the guy who let himself be dragged through the woods for twelve hundred miles by a dog. When I brought up Eric Weihenmeyer, the blind adventurer who had recently climbed Mt. Everest, Cliff referred to him as "the blind guy who the sherpas pretty much carried up the mountain."

After a few more sessions in which I returned home feeling down on myself and hopelessly frustrated with my disability, I was pretty sure that things were going from dubious to worse. Why was this relationship heading in a downward spiral? What strange dynamic was in play?

For an outside perspective, I asked Jessica, home for the summer, to spend a session with Cliff and me. But I felt somewhat nervous that the dynamic I had described to her would not emerge in the presence of a third party. Jessica told me to just relax. She was anxious to attend a session with me for her own benefit. She wanted to learn as much about mobility instruction as she could in order to help me throughout the summer days that lay ahead.

As our session in the local school gymnasium wore on, Cliff and I were doing fine together. My theory of the third party presence seemed to be correct. Nothing demeaning or snide had left Cliff's lips. As we walked down the hallway toward the parking lot, I felt crest-fallen. All the anecdotes I'd relayed to Jessica were just stories, amusing or annoying, take your pick. They weren't real unless they had been witnessed, verified. As Cliff held the door open for Jessica and me, he casually asked what I'd done over the weekend. I told him that I'd helped my mother paint a section of our old house. I explained how I could feel each clapboard with my brush. I had been able to take long, flowing strokes using my other, latex-protected hand as a border. I added that it had meant so much to me to feel like I was, once again, useful, that I had provided genuine help on a job that needed doing. I also added that my mom was impressed with my performance with the paint brush and my ability to work out a method that worked for me. I could feel myself grin at the remembering of it and was a little embarrassed at the obvious pride I'd revealed. But so what— so often as a blind individual you have no choice but to sit on the sideline of life. It's hard to know what's going on and even when you do, you can offer little to lend a hand.

How could I know that this turned out to be the perfect set-up. Cliff just couldn't resist. Maybe he reacted to the pride in my voice, but he swiftly retorted in a matter-of-fact tone, "Well, you know, Neil—an elephant can paint."

His remark brought me up short, and I experienced one of those moments of stunned silence. I didn't know how to respond because I had no idea what he was talking about.

But my big sister spun into action. "What's that supposed to mean?"

Cliff tried to defend himself by explaining that if you put a paintbrush in an elephant's trunk, it would paint on a canvas that was set up.

"What's your point, Cliff?" she shot back. "Do you think it's inspiring to compare Neil's achievement to an elephant's? Is that supposed to be encouraging or uplifting? Because, to me, and I'm sure to Neil, it sounds degrading!"

I never met with Cliff Shears again. I remember making the final decision while on the phone with Joe Stein. He asked me if I was sure I wanted to end my weekly sessions with Cliff because it could take some time to find another mobility instructor within commuting distance of my home. But I had thought it through, and while I knew I needed to learn the skills of maneuvering in my environment, I had to protect myself from anyone who caused me to routinely doubt myself or demean the fragile abilities I was attempting to nurture. I couldn't allow myself to be pummeled emotionally by someone who was supposed to build me up and help me prepare for tomorrow as a confident blind man. As technically good as Cliff probably was at his job, I had to feel that my teacher and I were on the same team and shared a common goal.

In the end, it took just a few weeks for Joe to hook me up with another mobility instructor, someone I came to love and respect and who returned those sentiments to me in full measure.

*a*I HAD MY DOUBTS THAT JOE would be able to find another mobility instructor at all. Vermont is rural, sparsely populated, and I had neither heard of nor met a professional mobility instructor in my life. But it happened. Joe phoned one day to tell Neil that he had found a newly trained mobility instructor, a young woman named Tracy Garland who lived not far from us. She worked for a Vermont-based, specialty food company that required her to travel for part of each week, but she was eager and able to take on a mobility client as well.

I think Neil and I were somewhat nervous on the day Tracy came to introduce herself. It's hard not to second guess yourself after making a decision that seems to surprise others. I was well aware that Cliff was a highly trained mobility instructor who helped a lot of people, people who were apparently glad to work with him. But Neil was clear in his own mind, and throughout the days following his decision, my late mother's voice reverberated deep within me: "There's no accounting for chemistry!"

When I opened the door to Tracy that first day, my anxiety ebbed. I felt myself open to one of those inexplicable moments of life, a moment that's just pure and uncomplicated. Standing before me was a cute, tom-boyish looking young woman in athletic clothing. She gave me a shy smile and I knew, immediately, that she, too, was a little nervous. I smiled back with the acknowledgment that she was the one we were waiting for.

*n*TRACY AND I HIT IT OFF from the very beginning of our relationship. She was the complete opposite of Cliff—encouraging and uplifting. She became excited when I made even small breakthroughs in my mobility skills. One day when we were out practicing together I slowed down to a near halt upon hearing a car idling ahead of me in a driveway, blocking the sidewalk as it waited to enter traffic. This feat—employing my hearing to navigate—induced Tracy to break into a song of praise, something she was prone to do after a challenging, could-be-dangerous experience was behind us. Her positive spin instilled confidence in me, made me more available to learn. If there were areas where I was slow to learn, Tracy never made me feel small or unworthy. She was a natural teacher. She knew when to push me to focus harder and when to remain quiet and let me figure out how to make a correction or to change a tactic on my own.

We became good friends. I was always happy to be in Tracy's company and was eager to learn what she had to teach me. Often on our training outings we'd work our way into a cafe, have a cup of coffee together, sit and talk and laugh about life in general like two regular patrons out for a morning cup of joe. Then, after our brief hiatus, she would transform, seamlessly, from a good friend back into the role of my well-respected instructor as we began the final leg of our journey.

The fact that Tracy, invariably, expressed the same amount of pride in my accomplishments as I felt meant the world to me. She made me feel that, yes, learning to navigate in my new world would take time and perseverance, but it was within my reach. And I would not fail.

*a*NEIL AND TRACY WORKED TOGETHER ONCE a week for many months. They practiced on rural roads, on the bumpy sidewalks of Brattleboro, even on the steps of the downtown parking garage. Neil loved their lesson time and grew more confident. He became adept at maneuvering around the many wooden billboards which line our downtown sidewalks but still had major difficulty staying in a straight line at crosswalks, often veering too close to the traffic stopped for crossing pedestrians. Neil had learned the basics, but just as we discovered in the study of braille, there were deeper levels beyond, levels that were incrementally and fundamentally harder than the first tentative, promising steps.

Of course I wanted Neil to practice in between his weekly sessions with Tracy. It didn't always happen, but when he and I did plan an outing in order for him to practice, I could see how much bravery it took to even try navigating the world outdoors without vision. Sidewalks were studded with driveways that interrupted the edge of grass he tracked with his cane. Garbage cans, waiting to be taken in, had blown sideways across our path. Low hanging branches were waiting to suddenly smack his face. The cement underneath our feet often jutted upward as the result of frost heaves from the winter before. The crosswalks downtown made a chirping sound to call forth pedestrians, but they did so for a mere moment before they switched to the visual digital sign indicating the number of seconds remaining before the traffic would start up. In winter patches of ice threatened to send him crashing to his knees or his butt. The overwhelming roars of passing logging trucks, cement trucks, fire engines, motorcycles, and school buses made him jumpy. I could feel Neil's vulnerability even as I tried to calmly assert that the scary sounding vehicles were simply passing us and posed no threat. After a while, the concentration it took on Neil's part to make his way would lead to fatigue, and we would resume sighted guide for the remainder of our outing.

Eventually, Tracy's primary job took her out of state permanently. Her relocation was sad for both of them, but we did not seek another mobility instructor. Neil had learned the basics, knew what he had to do on his own to move forward. No one could really deal with the fear factor but him. He could choose to practice on his own or with a friend or family member at his back, but he seemed to drift into plateau mode in that area of independence. Being the social being that he is, Neil seemed to prefer going downtown or walking a country road with a friend at his side. And eventually he met Laura, his closest friend and kindred spirit, who traveled the streets of Brattleboro in her wheelchair. They formed a close bond which included jaunting around town together, he at the back of her wheelchair pushing when needed and she steering to their destination, the two of them chatting the whole way. They are a unique pair in town, each making up for the other's disability and a testament to creative ingenuity.

*n*WHEN I FIRST MET JOE STEIN, the timing wasn't good, but, in retrospect, could it ever have been? I was unable to get past the sickening probability that I was destined to stare into darkness forever, deprived of the visual beauty the world offered to everyone else. It overwhelmed my mind and my originally strong spirit, both of which had been derailed so suddenly and completely. I was unable to relate to actually being a blind person, living a life that revolved around white canes, braille, and talking computers. These were things for legitimately blind people, and I didn't want to be included in that group. I wasn't prejudiced toward the blind; I'd never even met a blind person—and, hey, I loved the musical masterpieces of Stevie Wonder and Ray Charles. Nevertheless, I'd always felt sad for them, being unable to see their enthusiastic fans who flocked to hear them sing and delight in their magical presence. Watching Stevie being led onto the stage before a performance, did I not think of his dependence as a sad limitation?

As for myself, how could I imagine a life not driving around town to take in the sights, not being able to watch the seasons change, never again seeing the faces of my loved ones? How could I live being so removed from the physical world, knowing it only by touch, a pathetic substitute for knowing it by sight? And now, what I perceived as Stevie's nightmare was mine as well. I had become part of an unfortunate population that I was not prepared to join. So I did the only thing I could—I fought it.

When Joe Stein visited me at home for the first time, I wasn't much different than I'd been at the rehab center—despondent and uncommunicative. I let him regale me with possible services but had no questions to show any interest in what he was offering. In keeping with our first meeting, my unwillingness to engage and my lack of affect did not dampen his kindness toward me. He wanted me to know that he was here to help, that he was confident that he could, and that things would start to fall into place with time.

As my parents showed Joe to the door that day, I heard my mother explaining that I was still coming to terms with my condition. I clenched my jaw and gritted my teeth. I felt as if this was a small betrayal. My own parents were resigned to the fact that I was permanently blind. I listened to Joe assure them that this was totally normal, that he was not offended in the least, and that he really looked forward to providing me with the services that would help me rebuild my life. When my parents rejoined me in the kitchen they simply hugged me and told me that although it didn't seem like it now, the days ahead would be better—that things would be all right. I hugged them back, grateful that they didn't mention my impolite behavior. And I hugged them for the energy they rallied every day in my behalf. But I bit my tongue in order to refute their false assertion. Because I knew beyond a doubt, as I had on that afternoon with Irving, that nothing in this dismal life I got would ever be all right.

～

My immediate family, through the grace of some higher spirit and their unequaled love for me never left my side during the sometimes tortuous steps of my rehabilitation. For the array of others who guided me in those early days I will always be grateful. And I fully acknowledge now, after having gained some distance from the pain of my losses, that I would not be where I am today if it were not for the support of Vermont Division for the Blind and Visually Impaired.

NINE

SOCIALLY SPEAKING

Don't walk behind me; I may not lead.
Don't walk in front of me; I may not follow.
Just walk beside me and be my friend.

\- Albert Camus

*a*IT DIDN'T TAKE LONG AFTER BEING released from rehab and taking up residence in his childhood home for Neil to realize that more than just his vision had been lost, more than his once good health had abandoned him. Just as demoralizing, just as sad, were the loss of friends who had been major players in his life when he could barrel down a mountain bike path, water ski behind a roaring motor boat, climb up through the rafters of a barn to patch the roof, throw and catch a Frisbee.

There were so many "guy things" that his life had revolved around, a type of being in the world that provided social engagement, self-definition, pride, and fun. There were times when Neil felt abandoned by old friends whose lives went on without him. And, of course, everyone's life does and must go on. This we acknowledged without bitterness, but the sorrow and loneliness for him and the wrenching grief for me, on his behalf, could not be denied.

The players who faded from his life did not, of course, "abandon" Neil. It's just that blindness had altered Neil so radically that their former shared activities and work experiences didn't fit anymore. Yes, there were drop-in visits and dinners out, but those were not the daily routines of the life they had once shared. Often, in response to an expression of nostalgia and defeat, I'd say to Neil, "Everything has changed now. And not everyone has the ability to adjust. Really, what you need are new friends—friends who have never known you differently than you are right now. And, with time, that will happen. I know it will." And he would agree, but the sadness for what had been could not be cast off by possibilities that lay in the distant future.

*n*EVERYONE WANTS PEOPLE IN THEIR LIVES they can depend on but the blind depend on others to such an extent it can cause stress and alienation in those you thought had your back, eventually separating you, regardless of your past history. More than once, I've had to face the reality that my dependence, my reliance on someone had gone too far. After the fact, it's very hard not to blame myself; couldn't I have given the person just a little more space?

Sometimes I can't help but think of myself as a burden, a wet blanket that a sighted person has to tow around. After a while it doesn't matter how great my attitude is, how funny I am, how downright handsome I am, I feel like a big unwieldy piece of luggage. The bottom line is that friends and acquaintances can step up to the plate for you now and then, but the resources needed to support a blind person on a daily basis are above and beyond what most people can offer. That extra mile can wear a friend or relative out and cause resentment. No one wants it to happen, but it can. I get it. From my perspective, however, it feels hard to be resented for something that is so obviously out of my control.

Oftentimes it's the little things— "Can you read me the directions on this pizza box?" Not such a big deal, but the little things add up. I've become pretty tuned in to the reality that people have very different capacities to cope with a friend's or loved one's limitations, especially one as significant as the loss of vision. It has been one of the most difficult, depressing elements of the life I got.

a TO THIS DAY, NEIL CHERISHES THE ones we still call the angels, who stuck by him throughout that first turbulent year, who made the adjustment to his new existence, who included him in their lives. Not a week went by in which the Hansen sisters, often with their parents, did not spend time with him in their homes or out and about. They laughed, they had conversations both lighthearted and deep, they shared joys and troubles and just "were" together.

George, old enough to be Neil's dad but eternally a kid, lonely himself and going through a divorce, had Neil over for dinner at least once a week. Neil would bring the fixings, and together they would concoct a meal. Afterward, they would often play the djembe drums together. Rich from down the road was also a generation older but one of the friendliest and most compassionate guys on the planet. He wanted to spend time with Neil on Monday mornings. They walked together, tandem biked, went out in a boat, and Rich experienced his first massage as one of Neil's volunteer subjects on a Friday morning in Chloe Grant's studio. Em and Robyn, Annie and Matt, all from the Greenwood School, kept in close touch, as did Seth, out in Colorado. Adam and Sue, a couple Neil knew from his days at the University of Vermont, and Neil's high school friend Emma, all living in Burlington, invited him to spend weekends to attend special events. Jesse, Neil's compadre from the University of Redlands who haled from Marin County, California, invited him to visit for a week. I couldn't believe that Neil, newly blinded, not that independent, and enduring chemotherapy would consider going to California, but he insisted on it. While there Neil convinced Jesse and Jesse's brother Beau to go skydiving. Yes—they all jumped out of a plane one afternoon in northern California. These angels, along with several friends he'd grown up with in Westminster West village, stayed the course with him, each in their own way.

Now, as the years have passed, many of them play very minor roles. Their lives have moved in different directions and Neil's has too. It's no different from the way life flows for all of us. But to each, we are indebted. We hold them in our hearts with love and gratitude.

WHILE A NUMBER OF PEOPLE I CONSIDERED my closest friends faded from my life when I became blind, others emerged to fill that void which contained such immense pain for me. I can never thank these precious souls enough for remembering me and caring for me during those days of confusion and loss.

One of the first to step up was George who I'd lifted weights with and worked with during my teen-age summers at the Putney School. I'd known him nearly my whole life. During my Year of Healing, I would wait for George on the front porch of my parents' house, holding a bag of fixings to prepare for supper. I spent countless evenings at his house, doing all I could to help prepare our meal while we both grooved to our shared love of reggae music booming from his massive sound system. Rich, a fellow Westminster West resident who had Monday mornings off from work, took me out for breakfast each week at The Front Porch Cafe in nearby Putney. I got a kick out of the fact that as I was no longer gainfully employed, I could actually look forward to Monday mornings! How could I not feel a rush of pleasure as I entered the cafe where everyone, especially the owners, knew me and were happy to see me? In my former life I had been a regular, devoted customer. Now I took pride in showing the world that despite what they had heard, I was back on my own two feet.

During my time at Greenwood I'd become close friends with Em, a teaching colleague, and her partner Robyn. Both women were warm and friendly and had been eager to bring me into the fold of campus life at Greenwood. I appreciated their different personalities—Em was "out-there," boisterous, funny, and fun; Robyn was shy, soft-spoken, steady, and calm. Both of them were heartsick about my troubles and my departure from Greenwood. During my Year of Healing they were a steady presence in my life. We went out for dinner, shopped, laughed, and carried on much as we had at Greenwood. While Em maintained a full schedule of teaching and extra-curricular activities at the school, Robyn was between jobs.

While I had it in my head, initially, that I could get friends to pick me up and take me to my weekly schedule of therapy sessions, massage appointments, and whatever else popped up on my calendar, my mother and my Aunt Sali convinced me that that would not always be possible. The unreliability of depending on friends with busy lives would cause stress for us and add undo pressure on those relationships. They believed that in order for the year ahead to run smoothly, I should hire a driver who had a flexible schedule and pay him or her by the hour. And my mother had the perfect person in mind—Robyn. I could see that it would, in fact, be a win-win situation. I enjoyed Robyn's company, and she needed work. The idea became a reality almost immediately: Robyn, my friend, became my driver for the year.

As it turned out, Robyn and Em were in the process of searching for a new vehicle. The rural dirt roads leading up to the Greenwood campus could be challenging during winter as well as during what we Vermonters call "mud season" when the roads thaw. The car they shared was not four-wheel drive. The fact that they were in the market for a car lead to another (sort of) win-win situation.

One of the cruelest consequences of my blindness was the knowledge that I would never drive again. And an offshoot of that cruelty was saying good-bye to my beloved Nisson X Terra. I ended up selling it to Em and Robyn. I'd never be able to drive it again, but at least I could be an appreciative passenger and work the five disc changer like I was well practiced in doing. It made me happy to witness how excited they were with their new wheels, even if they could not fully feel the unimaginable pain the transaction brought me.

In any case, Robyn and I formed a close relationship. We had a fine time laughing and sharing just about anything that came up for either of us as we made our weekly rounds. And often, for the heck of it, we'd go out to lunch or dinner, simply because we wanted to hang out longer.

DESPITE THE HIGHS THAT THESE COMMITTED friendships brought to Neil's life, the lows were low enough to threaten me like a thunder cloud overhead, blocking any light I may have basked in for a stretch. The morning following the first party Neil attended after his homecoming, he described how uncomfortable and out of place he had felt in a setting that I knew once highlighted his social ease and grace.

When you are blind you cannot make the rounds in a crowd, mingle with ease, decide how long to engage in conversation and when to move on. When you are blind at a party you are either plunked in a corner like a coat rack or relegated to a couch, akin to one of the pillows that decorate it. People come up to you for greetings and conversation, but how awkward is it when they want to move on without their feeling they are abandoning you? And you sit, pretending to look perfectly content, until someone else happens by. All you can be is passive.

The same thing happened when I invited Neil to my students' annual spring concert. I knew he'd enjoy the music, would applaud with gusto from his seat in the audience, might get a kick out of attending a performance so similar to the ones he had sung in when he was their age. He knew the kids in my class. He had been coming into my classroom regularly to work with the students in ways that he was able. Why wouldn't he attend their concert?

The concert, itself, was pleasurable to Neil, but it was the pre-concert situation and setting that highlighted his disability in such a raw and predictable way. Our class was told to gather in the library to await each member's arrival. We would then be called by loud speaker to proceed to the auditorium to take our assigned place on the stage. I brought some magic markers and games for kids to engage in while we waited. But, of course, they were in high spirits, noting each others' dress up clothes and heady about being together during evening hours. Most of them greeted Neil in the way we had taught them, "Hi, Neil, it's Amy!" so that he knew who had approached him and could respond back, using their names.

But that was the extent of all interchanges during our wait. He could not comment on their outfits, could not look at their drawings, could not spot the boys who were running around and intervene by saying, "Come here buddy and chill with me while we wait"—things that would have been natural and easy for the original Neil, the charismatic guy who could slip into an authoritative role without turning anyone off.

I sized up the scene in that room immediately, knowing that there was nothing I could do to change it, to make it less awful for Neil as he sat alone in the center of the hubbub but completely disconnected from the flow of it.

We talked about the concert on the way home. I cannot recall whether he enjoyed the kids' singing, felt good about his post-concert chitchat with the teachers who had known him and taught him years before. All I remember is the pain he expressed from the waiting room experience—his feelings of uselessness, of isolation, of grief.

I told him that I heard him, that his pain was my pain, that I'd realized right away that the venue was a poor choice on my part. I was calm and supportive and I held it together. But as we drove I could feel that choke hold of despair asserting itself again—squeezing the life out of whatever happiness and hope I was trying to nourish within.

∼

Mia faded from our lives several months after Neil was released from rehab. I say "faded" because her disengagement from Neil was not abrupt. There was no official break-up, no declaration that the relationship had run its course, no sad or hurt good-byes.

My take on it is this: she and Neil, both in survival mode, both trying to grasp the reality of what had happened, unable to picture how the future would play out for either of them, were not equipped to express their fears and doubts to each other. Mia gave it a shot, did the best she could, I'm sure. But in the end, she pulled away.

I watched it happen. Always on guard, hyper-alert for trouble, I noticed how she became reluctant to linger and chit-chat with Jim and me. One day as she and Neil and I were finishing a meal at a nearby cafe, she announced her intention to drop in on a friend as soon as we were through. Neil spoke up, "Hey, mind if I come along?" For a nanosecond she hesitated. It was the tiniest blip that no one would have felt or noticed but me. Almost instantaneously she answered, "Of course!" But I knew— she had revealed in that tiny pause—that she didn't really want Neil to accompany her.

I could feel my heart harden. I felt the betrayal on my son's behalf. Mia would not stay the course. Her love for Neil was attached to the guy he had been and the future life she had envisioned for them as a couple. True, her plans and dreams had been torn away from her, one trauma after another during the agonizing weeks of his diagnosis, his surgery, his physical decline, and the ultimate shock of his blindness. But what is love worth if conditions are stronger?

While I deeply resented Mia for her ultimate desertion of Neil at a time when he needed every support available and for denying him the sense of closure I felt he deserved, how could I blame her? What would I have done in her place? It was a question I simply couldn't answer. While my own love was unwavering, my support, without question, I was, after all, Neil's mother—had brought him into this world with a kind of divine pledge that we would be connected to each other forever. If I was required to take on the role of caregiver, like it or not, I would, without hesitation. But would I be able to do that for someone who was not my flesh and blood or for whom I had not yet "pledged my troth?"

Mia and Neil were not married. They had endured storms in their relationship once the initial infatuation of their early dating had passed. Mia was practical, organized, serious about where she was headed, and was tied to a life of responsibility to her family. Neil was fun-loving, carefree, creative, impetuous, and somewhat spacey. They loved and admired each other's qualities. They needed the balance that the other brought into their life together, but their combination of opposites could drive the other crazy. They had broken up once already prior to Neil's crisis and, like so many couples, had reunited because they were lonely and missed each other. They missed "having someone."

When Neil was first released from rehab and took up residence at our home in Westminster West, I would regularly drop him off at the house Mia shared with her dad, and he would spend the night and try to renew the life they'd had. One hot, humid day, Mia had suggested they take the short hike from her house to the woodland creek where they had loved to frolic. When I picked Neil up the next day prior to Mia's shift at the hospital, he told me that the jaunt had been a complete bust. While Mia had done her best to lead him over some rough terrain, he kept stumbling, tripping, hurting himself in one way or another, and when they got there, he couldn't handle the mosquitoes that bit him relentlessly. If only he had been able to see, he was sure he could have swatted at least some of them. He admitted to me that, basically, he complained and whined the whole time. As he recounted all the discomforts of the experience, I couldn't help but imagine how awful the trip to the creek had been for Mia and what a sad contrast it must have been to previous memories of their times there together.

In her behalf, Mia gave their altered life ample chance to see if she could adjust. I believe she was working with a therapist during those months to process the trauma she had endured, perhaps to address, as well, the inevitable guilt of extricating herself from our lives—Neil's life and the life of our family which had been important to her. I imagine it must have been terribly painful and that she must have felt sad and alone. But, in the end, she made her choice.

As the years have passed, Neil has crossed paths with Mia now and again, and her father stops to visit him from time to time. Neil says, "I will always love Mia because she saved my life. She was the one who insisted I see a doctor when I was having those weird symptoms." And I tell him, "You know, Neil, sometimes angels come into your life to guide you when you need them. But they're not meant to stay. They aren't meant to be part of your life for the long haul. They go their own way, embark on their separate journeys."

And so it is with Mia. Neil has no regrets that they did not stay together. Both of us wish her the good life she deserves. I feel great compassion for all that Mia endured so bravely and gratitude that, for a time, she and I were comrades on the same team.

*m*MIA AND I PARTED WAYS THE YEAR I lived with my parents and underwent treatment. The abrupt change from the man I'd been to my diminished and overwhelmingly needy new self in those earliest days of my blindness must have been over-whelming for her. I can only imagine her shock, her grief, and, eventually, her frustration. I had become a pathetic little pawn in the game of chess, requiring careful maneuvering around my environment. To watch someone you loved— who you had counted on to make elaborate, sophisticated moves like the dominant queen or the formidable horse—become so reduced must have been a source of great confusion and pain for Mia. But we could never really talk about it or come to terms with it one way or another.

A particular night sticks out in my memory as pointedly as my ribs did from my wasted physique in those days. I was staying with Mia at her father's New Hampshire farmhouse where she had taken up permanent residence after earning her nursing degree. I awoke in the middle of the night having to use the bathroom. And I knew this was going to be a big deal for me. Unlike my parents' house, Mia's had not in any way been made "user-friendly" for a guy with no sight. And now, because of the call of nature, I had to circumnavigate the unfamiliar placement of furniture and piles of who knows what lying helter-skelter on Mia's bedroom floor.

Mia had embarked on a summer of projects, and it seemed to me that random objects were piling up all around the place making the house more cluttered than it used to be. I was pretty sure this wasn't just my imagination at work, and I wondered at the coincidence of it. Was it really necessary that she embark on elaborate home improvement projects this particular summer— the summer following my brain surgery— on a house that hadn't had anything done to it for at least two decades? And I'm not talking about a couple days of leisurely painting in the neediest of rooms. All of a sudden, three generations of wallpaper had to be scraped from the ancient plaster walls of most of the rooms. Mia spent hours using a caulking gun, a skill I had taught her about a year before, in my "sighted" days, as I began referring to them. And now she went about meticulously filling cracks in the walls and ceilings.

As I silently planned my course of action, I could feel Mia's calm, even breathing as she slept beside me. I did my best to envision the floor plan of the bedroom, a room I'd known well but couldn't have imagined I'd ever need to memorize. As my flood gates were giving a warning signal, I knew it was time to make my move, and I had a plan. I would use the walls to guide me through the bedroom and down the hallway to the bathroom.

I swung my feet to the floor and pushed off from the bed. My hand touched the nearest wall. I was neatly sandwiched between the wall and the mattress and felt pretty confident. I inched my way to the foot of the bed and turned the corner. "I'm doing damn well," I thought, proud that I hadn't made a sound. I felt a happy surge for this feat of independence. I let go of the foot of the bed and took two tentative steps, using only this new wall to guide me now. And then two more steps. It was late at night, obviously dark outside, and suddenly I felt free, just like a normal guy going to take a piss at night.

Using my new visualization skills I figured it couldn't be more than a couple of steps, so I took a large, bold, confident stride and was met with a deafening SMASH as I collided—no, crashed—into a large, metal object. I cracked my big toe so hard against the base of the object that I let out a sharp yelp. The collision threw me totally off balance sending me backwards a few feet. My seemingly successful, first independent run to the bathroom had been thwarted by—what? And then I remembered the industrial-sized floor sander that Mia had rented from Agway two days before. I remembered hearing her dad struggling to unload it from the back of his truck while I sat idly by.

Of course the sound of the collision woke Mia instantly. And it seemed that she must have been wakened from a terrible dream. It was the only explanation I could imagine for her fury towards me.

"Neil, what the hell are you doing?"

I was so shocked by the tone of her voice that I couldn't answer. I just stood there dumbly like a deer caught in the head-lights. My moment of bewildered silence seemed to fuel the fire of her rage against me. Was she still in a dream-like state? It became clear in the next moment, however, that she was fully awake, as she began to bark specific orders at me: "To the right, Neil—no—your other right, Neil!"

I couldn't get a clear idea of what I was supposed to do, which way I was facing, which way I was supposed to turn to get back on track, how far away the door was. And my befuddlement only made Mia more exasperated with me.

As fast as I dared, trying to escape the verbal tongue-lashing, I half limped and half awkwardly shuffled the remaining short distance to the bathroom. I closed the door, located the toilet and lowered myself down, the way I was becoming accustomed to right after I'd lost my sight and, with it, my accurate aim. As I let the urine flow, I gingerly felt for my big toe. I could feel a warm liquid, obviously my own blood, ooze from under the nail. I tore off a long piece of toilet paper and wrapped my toe like a mummy. It was already throbbing.

I sat on that toilet for what seemed a long time, my mind throbbing as well. I felt as though I was all alone in an inhospitable place. And a new goal replaced the one I'd nurtured earlier—the goal of doing my duty without rousing my girlfriend from her slumber. I longed to be in a familiar, comforting environment. I just wanted to go home. I felt utterly defeated as well as abandoned by someone who had once loved me, and the last thing I wanted to do was attempt the return trip to bed.

I did, in fact, make it to my side of the bed without incident, but I never fell back to sleep that night. I lay in the dark and finally connected the dots that practically connected themselves. It became clear why Mia showed such reluctance—actually refusal—to stay with me at my parents' home, despite the fact that my father had labored to turn the large, upper, front room into a cozy little efficiency, redoing the bathroom and fixing the outdoor staircase that ran from the driveway right up to what could have been Mia's and my own little apartment, complete with a little galley kitchen. But it hadn't mattered what efforts my folks had made to accommodate us as a couple, to make Mia feel at home or at least comfortable. No wonder why she consistently insisted on staying at her dad's. And it was no longer a mystery, in my mind, why she started all these overwhelming projects when she did. There was no longer room for me—the sightless me—in her life. Mia had no desire left to try to carry on. Whatever we'd had together was over. Otherwise, she would have shown a modicum of concern or compassion over my collision with the sander. But she hadn't. Instead, she had turned away and gone back to sleep. I spent the remaining hours coming to terms with the reality that I was swimming alone. I sank into a dark, private pool of my own thoughts regarding my failures and inadequacies. No matter how hard I kicked or stroked, it was a struggle to stay afloat, to keep my head above water. And no proverbial lifeguard was on duty to save me from myself.

In the end, and that end is actually hard to pinpoint, Mia stopped being part of my life. We were never able to process all that had happened and how it affected us as a couple. She just gradually stopped communicating, stopped making plans to spend time together. I understood that for her, and perhaps for both of us, this was easiest; the finality of bidding farewell to a three year relationship was too painful.

I will always have love in my heart for Mia. If it were not for her insistence, I probably wouldn't have discovered the tumor until it was too late. I've often imagined being alone in my Greenwood apartment and going into massive, continuous seizures with no intervention. How can I not feel an immense debt and just as much gratitude to her?

Every March, with some sadness in my heart for all we endured together, I call Mia on her birthday and tell her voice mail that I am thinking of her and am so thankful for every day that I am alive and that I have her, in part, to thank. I hope that she, too, wakes up on her birthday feeling that it's the most magnificent day!

~

People have asked me what it's like to be blind. When the subject comes up, most sighted people express the opinion that it must be way better to have seen the world before becoming blind than never having had the opportunity at all. After giving it some thought, I'd have to say I agree. I am eternally grateful for all I got to see in the twenty-eight years that I was blessed with sight: beautiful women, the glory of nature, the Patriots scoring a touchdown at the last second, my mother's gorgeous face, a bright red Ferrari, oh so sleek—and, yes, I did say red, because I know what colors are. Memories of these images bring me joy. I thank the spirits of life, or a higher being, for my ability to see them, still, in my mind's eye, if not with my actual eyes.

A well-known line from a Joni Mitchell song— "Bettcha

don't know what you got 'till it's gone!"—brings up the flip side of becoming blind later in life, and that is the sorrow and heartbreak of it all. Had I been born blind I wouldn't experience the excruciating sadness of listening to cars pass by on their way to wherever their drivers please, quick as a breeze. I might not be immersed in isolation, sitting in the background as a friend hits a home run at the annual softball game, wishing it was me and knowing it never will be. I wouldn't long, with all my heart, to be included in the group of people marveling at how beautiful the sunset is while I stare dumbly into nothingness.

Blindness is a cruel disability. I'd read at one time that ninety percent of the human brain's intake is from the visual sense. I never thought that I'd ever have first-hand experience to corroborate this statement, but I do, and I agree. I am, so much of the time, on the outside of human experience, and I know it. I know it because I didn't used to be.

And then there's the fear factor that others never know. It's impossible for me to be aware of everything that I'm missing—all the vital information that kept me safe, enabled me to be a highly functioning individual. Outside of the small comfort zone that is my home, my street, my block, it becomes an entirely different ballgame. When I'm in an unfamiliar place, my surroundings are completely alien. I admit to sometimes having nightmare-type thoughts in public places, even while I'm sitting comfortably among friends or acquaintances. I imagine that the fire alarm suddenly goes off, and everyone runs out of the building in a panic, leaving me behind in a completely unfamiliar room I had been led into.

I don't stand a chance. I have no clue of where the doors are or which direction to turn, but I frantically search for an exit with my cane, smashing into everything as the flames lick up around me.

It has been difficult beyond measure coming to terms with the fact that I live in a state of hyper-vulnerability that I would rather not share with others. The social aspects of not being fully aware of what is going on around me, being dependent on others for help, and not being useful or capable of helping others in return, whittle away at my pride and sense of self worth. These are the indignities I must endure and, somehow, make peace with.

TEN

TREATMENT

May you always be courageous,
stand upright and be strong.

~ Bob Dylan

BECOMING BLIND OVERNIGHT WOULD PROBABLY rate among the top nightmares for most of us. And yet Neil's situation had a weird, murky, silver lining: dealing with blindness is so all-encompassing that the daily challenges kept us from obsessing about the fact that he had a very serious form of cancer. That part of our reality paled in comparison to his coping with living in a dark and confusing world. One day in the car Neil said to me, "I can't believe I have cancer," and I responded, "Me neither." The cancer simply did not have the power over us it would have, had it been the main focus.

I used to think that if one of my children was diagnosed with cancer, I would not be able to bear it. I'd curl into myself like a dry November leaf, paralyzed by fear and grief. But making our way during those early days at home, I barely thought about it. There simply wasn't room in a mind overloaded with the continual task of figuring out how to manage the next half hour in uncharted territory.

Yet there was a part of me that was aware that weeks were passing following Neil's diagnosis and surgery, and the treatment that would save his life was on hold. Dr. Renaud continued to assure me, however, that we were on track and that Neil was addressing everything he needed to prior to radiation and chemo. His full year of treatment would happen in short order, and the wait did not bode ill for the outcome.

Neil began treatment for his brain cancer in the late spring of 2008, about three months following his diagnosis and surgery. The plan was to undergo six weeks of radiation, five days a week, at Southside Medical Center. Immediately following radiation he would undergo twelve rounds of chemotherapy with regular monitoring by Dr. Renaud at University-North. The parameters of our life were set. In addition to the challenges of learning how to cope with blindness, Neil now needed to address the business of staying alive by carefully following medical schedules.

Often that year I thought about how bad it was that Neil had cancer. And then I thought about how horrible it was that he had to live the rest of his life in darkness. And then I thought how absolutely intolerable it was that he had to deal with both. I wished that Neil could be just one or the other, cancer patient or newly blinded individual. But which would I even choose for him? Of course I knew it was an impossible and ridiculous question. What was the point of even musing on such a choice, as if we mortals possessed the power to rewrite reality? But sometimes I couldn't help myself. We are, it seems, hard wired with imagination that attaches itself to longing. And that powerful combination can box us into some strange corners.

~

If I can label Neil's situation lucky in any way, it would be the manner in which his body and psyche handled the barrage of radiation and chemicals that were rained upon him. He had several advantages: he was young, he exercised daily, he'd been strong and healthy his whole life. Along the pathway of his growing up, as a spirited youth eager to explore a life of his own design, I knew he'd abused his body in pretty predictable ways: too much alcohol, too much marijuana, too much junk food. But his body had tolerated poor choices. It was at the peak of its own divine cycle. It was forgiving of the reckless driver at the controls and bounced back dutifully, cheerfully even, from short-sighted neglect. Like most people his age, Neil had taken his health for granted. But now, suddenly, the game had changed. Neil was being asked to—and there really was no choice in the matter—kick his body in the guts, poison it on purpose, ask it to forgive him, and count on it doing so regardless of the hits it was being forced to withstand. It was a tall order.

We read all the brochures about possible and probable side effects of the radiation, then later, the chemo. The journey he was about to embark on felt like an anti-adventure. It was a supreme test. But at least we'd done our best to familiarize ourselves with the road map.

∼

Neil's six weeks of radiation treatment had a science-fiction-y air about it, requiring the use of a macabre mask, a mapping technique designed to locate the exact position of the tumor, and a powerful beam which released a zap with pinpoint precision. The most graphic part of the whole ordeal was the making of the mask that would be laid over Neil's face and firmly fastened to the table on which he lay, ensuring that no movement on his part could deflect the beam from its target. The process of making the mask required him to lie flat on his back while plaster of Paris was applied to his face. While still wet, a flexible sheet of screen which looked like garden variety window screen was sunk into the plaster and molded to his face. When it dried it was rigid yet soft. It looked just like Neil. He got the biggest kick out of it, couldn't wait for me to see it, and announced that he wanted to keep it as a trophy once it was retired from use. I laughed when he told me this. How could I not admire his playfulness and quirky intention while dealing with such serious and scary business?

One day when we arrived at the clinic for his appointment, the nurse was not yet back from lunch. The technician called out to us, "Come on back—I'm all ready for Neil!" I led him into the treatment room, made chit-chat with the technician who was now a "good bud" of Neil's, and watched as my son was positioned and locked down on the table, ready for his precision point zap. As I turned to leave, my eyes caught sight of a whole row of screen masks, all shaped exactly like their owners' faces, looking as though they were waiting dutifully for their owners' return. It was a very visual, very surreal moment for me. I turned and fled from what suddenly felt like a bizarre movie set.

The effect of the radiation treatment was cumulative over time. It took its toll on Neil in increasing fatigue as the days and weeks went by. After a session one beautiful spring day I told Neil I had to stop at the supermarket to pick up a few things. He was game. We grabbed a cart, me guiding the front, him pushing energetically from behind. We entered the store and made our way down an aisle. Ten minutes in I turned to ask him something and was shocked to see him completely changed from the person he'd been in the parking lot. He looked wilted, deflated, exhausted.

"Let's get out of here," I said. "I don't need anything more than what's in the cart already. Let's head home."

"Sounds good to me," he answered with a tired smile. Ten minutes after we pulled into the driveway he was in his bed, asleep.

*n*THAT DAY STANDS OUT FOR ME, as well. I remember feeling fine—energy to spare—as we made our way down the aisles, me pushing the cart at the handlebar end and Mom pulling and guiding from the front. Suddenly, without any kind of gradual warning, all the energy in my body seemed to melt and seep out through the pores of my skin. I could feel myself slump over the bar of the cart that I was now grasping for support. My forward movement must have slowed because my mother picked up on the situation in short order. After asking me a few questions to verify what was already obvious to her, we left the cart where it stood. She led me out to the car, telling me she'd be right back. As I fell into what felt more like unconsciousness than sleep, she returned to our abandoned cart and checked out. I wasn't aware of anything until we were back home in our driveway, and she gently shook me back to life in preparation for a real nap in my awaiting bed.

Although the effects of radiation were intense, the treatments lasted just six weeks, five days on and two days off like a regular work week. Anyone receiving radiation to the brain must undergo a preliminary step—the making of a plaster mask. As I lay on my back that first day, I was told that the procedure would feel a bit weird, but it wouldn't take long and would not interfere with my breathing. The technician placed a warm, moist cloth over my face, and I could feel him applying, then spreading the plaster over it. In about five minutes the soft cloth had hardened into an exact mold of my face. Despite having lubed me up with some sort of grease before the procedure, as he lifted the mask from my face I felt sure that my goatee was going with it! The week after this preparatory session, my radiation treatments began. My mask, which went beyond my face to encase the whole front of my head, was bolted to the table, making even a millimeter of movement impossible. This was of the greatest importance as the radioactive beam can kill healthy cells just as easily as it kills cancerous ones. Despite the careful aiming of the beam, I did end up with some unfortunate but tolerable permanent side effects. I've lost about twenty-five percent of the hearing in my left ear, which is not something I wanted to give up, being blind and all. I mean, come on—my blessed hearing is one of the only things left to me. But it's an annoyance I manage. On a lighter note, another side effect hardly worth mentioning as I inherited the Taylor gene for baldness anyway and already kept my hair incredibly short is that I lost some hair, permanently, above my temple at the site where the beam entered my head. Actually, I'm told that both my left eyebrow and my eyelashes on that side are sparser than on the right. So I'm a lopsided guy. But these were small prices to pay for the benefits radiation delivered in helping shrink my tumor.

*a*DESPITE THE ACCUMULATING FATIGUE, Neil made it through the six week course of radiation in good spirits. Each day at the clinic he chatted and joked with the receptionist, the nurses, and the technicians. He remembered their stories, inquired about the trip one just took, the new dog another was taking to training school, the grandkids who were visiting from out of state. This is the way he'd been all his life—a "people" person, quick and funny, a ray of sunshine who beamed into your life spreading good cheer even when he, himself, was hurting. I understood this part of Neil on the deepest level. He was acting the way he wanted to feel. He was being nurtured by others, receiving as well as giving. He understood how to take care of himself emotionally.

One day, as he emerged from the radiation room on the arm of one of his admirers, I said, "Neil, Jerry just came in and is sitting right next to me." Jerry was a man in his mid to late sixties who was also being treated for a malignant brain tumor. He was always nattily dressed when we saw him at the clinic, an unusual looking guy, and I realized that his wire mask was probably in the line-up the day I'd accompanied Neil to the zapping table.

"Jerry!" Neil responded, reaching out to feel for Jerry's hand. "Hey, man, I just got that table all warmed up for you!"

Of course, everyone laughed. How could you not?

Neil withstood the thirty sessions of radiation to his brain with optimism. He was on his way to reclaim his health, and if fatigue was part of the package, he accepted it without complaint. Two weeks following his final zap, the radiologist in Keene proclaimed that "things were going in the right direction." Those were exactly the words we wanted to hear.

~

While Neil was in the midst of his radiation treatments, he was invited to participate in the graduation ceremonies at the Greenwood School. He was touched and honored by the invitation. It had been difficult for many of his young charges when he disappeared without warning from their lives in the dorm, the classroom, and the gym. His students had worried about him, had sent him heartfelt cards and letters while he was in the hospital and rehab center, and had wondered if they would ever see him again. His story had been followed by many of the parents who had also written to him expressing their appreciation for his work with their sons and wishing him a full recovery.

Neil was to sit on stage with the faculty and present an award to one of the graduating students. In the Greenwood tradition, each graduate would receive a book from a faculty member who had been involved with him in a significant way, a book that would be special and meaningful to that particular boy. The faculty member would address the audience, share an anecdote about his or her honoree, and call him forward to receive his book. Neil, indeed, had had a special connection to the boy he was to honor that day. He was proud of his student's growth and success, both academically and personally, during the time he had worked with him. And he wanted very much to express himself well at the event.

As the time drew nearer and nearer, however, Neil grew extremely anxious about his speech and simply could not come to a place of serenity or peace about it. I watched his anxiety grow and began to feel that this was simply not the time to take on this particular challenge. I asked him if he would like to rethink his commitment to participate, given that he was in the middle of radiation treatment. But he was adamant that he go through with it. He had not expected to be honored and included. He wanted to show his gratitude, wanted to connect with the school once more, wanted to be part of the celebration.

I told him that in my work as a teacher there were many times I had to speak in front of groups and what helped me most was to write down what I wanted to say. I would read it aloud a few times, and then before I was to begin, I'd throw the notes away. I figured I'd remember the essentials, that if I left something out, it was OK, but in my experience, I always thought that a presentation given informally, from the heart, without continually looking down at notes was more effective, more powerful.

Not only did I believe this, but the cold fact of the matter was that notes would be of no use to Neil. Had Neil not been blind, I would have given him the same advice, but it would have been his call whether or not to have his notes on hand for moral support.

What we ended up doing was writing down what Neil wanted to say and recording it. The recording was simply a variation of my practice. Neil would listen to it as much as he wanted, then let it go. It would serve him well as a foundation for his heart-felt remarks. But Neil was stuck in a panic mode that was not really like him. His plan was to memorize, word for word, the whole little speech, an unrealistic and unreliable approach. He practiced and practiced. I certainly understood one level of his nervousness: he was still young and had had little or no call to stand in front of a large audience before. He was inexperienced. That, I got. What was not immediately clear to me was that his memory was being affected by taking radiation to the brain. He couldn't and didn't trust himself to hang onto the essential points of what he wanted to say should he take my advice and toss the notes after listening to them several times. Those points would have floated away, and he would be left with a mind empty of content. In his mind, memorizing verbatim was the only way he could handle the task.

I conferred privately with Jim: "What's going on with Neil?"

And his immediate response enlightened me: "What do you think?" he responded. "His brain is being temporarily fried by radiation."

The afternoon of the graduation was a perfect Vermont May day, dry, sunny, not too warm in the emerald fields surrounding the school or under the festive white tent. Neil looked thin but handsome on stage seated next to his dear colleague, Em. I was grateful that she had planned to take Neil under her wing that day. She would lead him to the microphone when it was his turn. Her bighearted warmth, her outgoing, take-charge nature was just what he needed, I told myself. I calmed my own nerves by reminding myself that we were among friends.

We found seats in the second row: Jessica, Jackson, Mia, Em's partner, Robyn, and I. The graduating students before us, ready to transition to either public or private high schools after their lives at the specialized Greenwood School, looked a little subdued, but proud, in their blazers and ties, feeling all eyes on them and reflecting back the embarrassment that every young teen feels in such formal situations.

"This might not be the most fun afternoon for me," I remember thinking, but it was, nonetheless, a privilege to witness and share the passage these young men had worked hard for and earned. And my own son had been an integral part of this community of learning. His stint had been brief, but he had left his mark. I did my best to push down the incredible sadness that welled up, that it had all ended this way, and allow my gratitude to take center stage for as long as I could maintain it.

When it was Neil's turn to present, Em led him to the podium, and the audience stood in unison to clap for him—for his work with the boys, for the nightmare he had endured, and for the uncertain future that lay ahead of him. It was very moving. Neil stood before them, receiving all the recognition and well wishes they bestowed from their hearts. Finally they sat. And there was a very long silence. Too long. Neil just stood there like a deer in the headlights, and my heart dropped into my gut. Somehow, however, after what seemed maybe longer than it really was, he got his bearings and began the speech he had so meticulously prepared and practiced. It went well briefly; he managed the beginning, and then he hit a wall. He stumbled over a few words, paused and said, "I can't remember what I was going to say." Someone from the audience yelled out, "You're doing great!" but that offer of encouragement, that gift of support was not enough to help him corral the words that had evaporated like ether from his befuddled mind.

I knew I had to help. I called up to him, "Neil, didn't you

want to tell about the time you and your student...you know...!"
His face broke into a grin and he called down to me, "Oh, yeah,"
and skillfully and humorously told the tale he had wanted to
share. When he finished his anecdote, he stumbled again. I
called up, "And don't you want to tell us the name of the book
you selected and why you chose it?"

As he finished, his student came forward and they embraced,
completely oblivious of the crowd in front of them. The boy's
eyes were shut as he leaned his head on Neil's shoulder, but I
know there wasn't a person present who didn't see the tears
glistening on the boy's cheeks.

It was over. Neil had done what he had set out to do, and
it didn't matter in the least that he had needed some prompting
to get through it. We all congratulated him and deemed it a
success. We were asked to stay and have a bite and visit with
everyone, but we couldn't wait to leave, especially Neil. We said
our good-byes and returned home to share the good news with
Jim who admitted he never could have made it through the event.

~

Many weeks later I was tidying the upstairs hallway of our house.
I was sick of skirting the accumulated piles and paper bags of
household objects that had been relegated there waiting to be
sorted and deposited to their rightful places. I opened one of
the bags, and there was Neil's wire screen mask, lying on its
side. I reached for it and a wave of revulsion swept over me. I
hated that thing—did not want to look at it or be reminded of

what it represented. I knew that Neil had wanted to keep it, but he had not mentioned it since that first day. What positive purpose could this relic offer him? And maybe he'd never think to ask about it. I made up my mind. If and when he brought it up, well, I'd just have to tell him that I threw it away in a very weak moment.

~

Most people whose cancer stories I had followed prior to Neil's case were required to take a chemo infusion in a hospital setting and spent several hours on "hook up" to receive it. In contrast, Neil's chemotherapy was administered in pill form. His bottles of Temozolomide pills, or "Temodar" for short, were sent from a dispensary and arrived on our front porch each month. The chemo pills were to be taken, along with an anti-nausea tablet, five days out of each month. The bottles came with ominous directions warning us never to handle the pills. The labels stopped short of displaying a skull and cross bones, but the warning sobered me to the reality of what Neil must endure to get the upper hand on this tumor. Nevertheless, every month I was grateful that Jim could simply tap the tiny pills into a cup and bring them to Neil as he was getting ready for bed. Neil could swallow them, go to sleep in his own bed, and come down to breakfast the next morning.

His reactions to the chemotherapy became predictable in some ways and unpredictable in others. Predictable was the fact that during the five days of taking the pills, he was totally fine and could carry on as usual. The following week, however, after the accumulated potency of five pills in a row, he was fatigued and needed more rest. The unpredictable aspect was that some months, during his tired time, he was simply tired. Other months, he seemed more spacey, more foggy, more forgetful, somewhat "off." And there was no predicting when that would happen—some months, yes, some months, no. The foggier cycles did not seem to occur due to a "build up" of the drug over the year's time. The condition would present itself in month four, for example, and not in month seven. There was no figuring. Eventually his head would clear, however, with no obvious lingering side effects.

*n*I BEGAN CHEMOTHERAPY ON THE HEELS of my radiation treatment. Luckily for me, the drug of choice for my particular tumor, a drug with the ability to cross the blood-brain barrier, came in pill form. Don't get me wrong—Temodar, like all chemotherapy, is a highly toxic concoction—and my body could sense it. Every time I swallowed the pills I had to restrain my gag reflex to keep from throwing them back up. I realized that a war would be happening inside me. I needed to ingest something highly poisonous in order to cure myself of something even more lethal. I was happy to be living with my parents, as the pills came in a variety of potencies which needed to be combined to make up my required dose. I remember thinking that you really had to have your head on straight to sort it all out, and I knew that mine was a little off-kilter during this time. Luckily, I was free from worry about messing up anything of that importance, as my father would come into my room with the proper dosage and a glass of water just as I was settling down for the night.

I took the Temodar pills for five days at the beginning of each month, then had a break for twenty-five days. And this schedule was repeated for twelve cycles—a full year. Temodar, because it is taken orally, has the reputation of being less fatigue-inducing than the intravenous route. I cannot speak from the perspective of someone who has experienced both, but I can say that if my journey was less fatiguing, then patients taking intravenous chemo must not get out a lot or even at all. While I did my five days of pill popping, I slept a solid twelve hours each night, and during the day I felt fine. But three or four days afterward, fatigue would sweep over me and invade every cell of my body. Even on short walks around the house I'd be overcome by a type of tiredness I cannot put into words. Sometimes, getting from the first floor up our long stairway to where my bed was waiting on the second floor seemed more than I could handle.

Aside from the long naps I needed during these times, I also suffered on and off from brain fog. My memory, which had always been strong, seemed to wither. I was routinely puzzled and would ask questions about something we had been discussing just minutes earlier. Likewise, I'd start to search frantically for something I'd misplaced, and in a matter of minutes I couldn't remember what I was looking for. I was left feeling disturbingly dim-witted. I'd test myself by trying to remember what I'd eaten for dinner the night before. It often took what felt like a good ten minutes of wracking my brain to recall the answer. When family or friends asked me questions during routine small talk, I'd sometimes make up something if I thought I could get away with it. This wasn't a plan I'd devised in advance. It was more like a split second decision born from the fact that my lack of simple cognition creeped me out and was hard to admit to.

a EACH MONTH THROUGHOUT THAT YEAR, Jim and I drove Neil to University-North to have his blood checked for stability or abnormalities, and every third time he would undergo a brain MRI to monitor how his tumor was responding to the Temodar. Waiting in Dr. Renaud's office on those third months was very trying, as any cancer family will attest to. It's hard not to go to the place of "will the ride home be happy or upsetting?" And you know that behind all the closed doors of all those other waiting rooms the same drama is cycling in other minds. It is not an easy way to live.

Eventually, Dr. Renaud would enter, computer under his arm and say, "It looks good!" Neil would cheer, and I would hug him, and Jim would squeeze my hand. Dr Renaud would proceed to show us the images of Neil's brain, comparing it to the time before. Yes, the ride home would be happy beyond happy. We were free and clear for another three months. Dr Renaud would proceed to give Neil a brief neurological check up, asking him to respond to simple muscle commands: "Push your legs against my hands; touch your finger to your nose; tell me if I am running my finger up your arm or down on your arm." Neil's brain to body connections were always intact. Finally, Dr. Renaud would check Neil's eyes, beaming a light directly into each pupil and peering in with his head practically touching Neil's head. With regard to Neil's vision, there was never change. But in Dr. Renaud's office that year there was banter, teasing, laughter, and general high spirits. Our happiness was his happiness; our suffering he met with compassion. Due to his cultural upbringing outside of this country, he was, by American standards, very affectionate, very touchy-feely with Neil, laying his hand on Neil's arm as he asked about what was going on in Neil's life, hugging him as they said good-bye. And what could be more affirming, more "connecting" for a blind person? In Dr. Renaud's presence, Neil felt truly cared for and cared about. Dr. Renaud was a natural. He "got it." And Neil, Jim, and I loved him for it.

AT THE OUTSET OF MY YEAR OF HEALING, Judy, my mother's closest friend and confidant, asked Mom if she was aware that the treatment I was about to undergo could render me sterile. She had done some research on the topic and had read that many young men who are faced with a course of chemotherapy choose to store sperm in the event that they decide to conceive children at a later date. Judy knew we were under tremendous emotional stress dealing with both my diagnosis and disability, but she said she'd feel remiss if she did not bring up the subject. Fertility was definitely not at the top of my triage list. Neither my family nor I had thought of it, and it had not been broached by my doctors.

My mother was appalled. As she shared with me what she had learned, we both acknowledged that although we wished I'd been told, my doctors were more than likely far more focused on my survival than on my down-the-road procreation. Luckily, and unbeknownst to me, I'd had Judy to cover third base. As luck would have it, I was scheduled to meet with Dr. Renaud the following day. When I brought the subject up, he assured me that he had known many men who had become fathers following cancer treatment. But he understood my concern and immediately scheduled an appointment at the fertility clinic at University-North. As my treatment was about to begin in four days time, I was jumped to the top of the list and was told to show up at the clinic the next day.

Although the issue of children had not made its way to the forefront of my mind—I was still floundering around trying to make my own way in the world, still learning to take care of myself—I had, from time to time, fantasized about the idea of having a family of my own. If that should happen, I planned to be the coolest dad on the block. Maybe, in the end, I would decide not to have children. But I wanted to have a choice.

On our way to the clinic the next day Mom did her best to get me to relax. She told me that whatever happened would be OK and that she loved me no matter what. As we drove, we chanted "Om Namah Shivaya" together, a chant we both loved, and, like always, it worked its magic on me. When we pulled into the parking lot, I felt as calm and relaxed as I possibly could. In short order we were sitting side by side in the clinic.

Before long, what sounded like a large male nurse greeted us in a deep voice and led us out of the waiting room and back to a smaller room, closing the door behind us.

"Hi, I'm Maude," came the deep, rich voice, again, "and I'll be right back."

This day was beyond weird, given where I was and what I had to do, and now I had apparently mistaken the gender of the nurse in charge of me. I felt as if I couldn't rely on anything within me to gain any kind of control of this situation.

"Mom, I whispered, trying to ground myself. "Is Maude a man or a woman?"

"Shh," Mom whispered. "A woman."

When Maude returned with whatever it was she'd forgotten, it was time for my mother to make her exit. As the door closed behind her, Maude began her rundown of the array of erotic material on hand. I heard her rifling around in a drawer and recognized the heavy thud that magazines make when they are stacked together, lifted and plopped down again.

Before I could interject, Maude added that many sperm donors prefer an erotic video and that she'd be more than happy to fire one up for me.

I stopped short. "Oh," I stammered. "I'm not actually a sperm donor. I'm here because I'm just about to start treatment for cancer, and any sperm I leave today will be saved for me if I ever need it." I added that since I was blind—had no sight at all—the magazines would probably do me little good and the same for the erotic film.

There was a moment of awkward silence before Maude excused herself from the room. In a few minutes another woman returned in the company of my mother. She introduced herself as Dr. Fitzgerald and apologized for their mistaking me for another male donor. I nodded my head and struggled to produce a faint smile. As she gave us a brief orientation regarding sperm saving, the only thing that stood out for me was the fact that two samples, deposited on different days, were required. I would have to return to the clinic once more before this ordeal was over. My mouth went dry, and I could feel a muscle on the good side of my face begin to twitch. Even if I was successful this first time around, which was seeming more and more doubtful, there was no getting out of a second run.

As my mother and the good doctor exited, Maude returned, giving me a strong sense of deja vu. Suddenly the confusion and anxiety I had been feeling inside myself receded for a moment, and I thought about poor Maude. Even if she had known I was blind, and I wasn't totally convinced this was the case, what more could she offer me from her treasure chest of erotica? How could anyone in her line of work veer from the usual protocol?

When she suggested the tried and true video again, I quickly agreed. This whole thing was weird enough for me; why should I make it even weirder for her? I figured, hell, I'm going to need all the help I can get, and possibly the audio aspect of the video— heavy breathing, a sultry female voice calling out, "Yes, Big Boy, that's the spot," or the simple, rhythmic slapping together of naked flesh—would do it for me. There was only one way to find out, I thought, as Maude pressed Play and bid me farewell and good luck. I was left alone in the dark, as always, leaning against a table for balance, holding an empty plastic cup in my left hand.

For years I'd invariably counted on my sexual response—it had never let me down—but under these circumstances I couldn't feel the slightest hint of it in my entire body. Even if Pamela Anderson or Heidi Klum walked in to take on the role as my sexy nurse assistant, it wouldn't have mattered, wouldn't have done any good. To round out this deteriorating scene, the recommended video had no titillating audio which I'd banked on to get me through this. All its sound track offered was heavy base notes in a frenetic pounding manner. If any situation could be less sexually evoking than trying to produce a sperm sample into a little plastic cup in a pitch dark hospital room in the inner sanctums of a fertility clinic while your mother waits patiently on the other side of a rather thin door, then, by all means, let's hear it. Couldn't I have foreseen this? How did I let this get so far? Was I really expected to ejaculate on command under these circumstances?

I had to try. I had to take this awkwardly orchestrated opportunity to pass my seed along into the vast ocean of human evolution. I owed it to the greater goodness of the world. At the very least, I owed it to my mom.

Using the table for balance, I removed my pants, placing them carefully beside me on the table so I could locate them by touch when I needed them. I slid my underwear down around my thighs. The table felt surprisingly chilly pressed against my naked butt. Here I was, fully exposed, to do the job I'd come here to do. As I assumed the position you can most likely picture, I gave myself a couple of gentle tugs of encouragement. I tried to think back to my last sexual experience. Was it at one of the last sleepovers at Mia's? I suddenly realized that I had not masturbated since I had learned about the tumor. Although I was well-trained in the art of pleasing myself in the past—I could do it in almost any location and pretty quickly—now under the current circumstances the whole thing felt foreign and bizarre. But I'd promised myself and the world that I'd give it a shot. I tried conjuring up all the most graphically erotic memories of my life followed by the lustful, tried and true fantasies that had served me so well in the past. On the physical level, I ran through my gamut of personal techniques and a few new ones to boot. Soft and gentle, vigorous and quick—nothing was working no matter how hard I tried. And I was running out of moves. My penis, like the rest of my pathetic body, was failing me. It had thrown in the towel with everything else.

After about ten minutes I became resigned to the fact that it was not going to happen. Feeling more that a little humbled, I hiked up my skivvies. I sat on the table for a few minutes feeling sorry for myself and putting off the inevitable sharing of my failure with what felt like the rest of the world, represented primarily by Maude. I located the office door and called out to my mother that I was done. And she called back, "Already?"

Obviously, Mom gave me more credit than I was due. With a tinge of shame I called back to her as quietly as possible that I simply could not do it. After a brief silence, Mom called back to me, also in a lowered voice, "Are you sure, honey?" I professed, sadly, that I was more than sure, and I asked her to come in and rescue me. I wanted nothing more than to leave this fertility clinic, this hospital, this whole day of my life behind me. I heard the door open, and my mom stepped into the room.

During all of my futile efforts, I had semi-forgotten about the porn flick, now playing out in all its graphic splendor in front of my mom. "Gross," I heard her say. "Neil, let's turn this thing off."

"Mom, I'm obviously not going to be much quick help here," I told her. "Just press Stop on the VCR."

My mother is less than technologically savvy, and being under pressure always makes her freeze. "I'm looking for that button—I can't find it—it's not marked," she retorted in an increasingly frustrated tone.

Three things went through my mind concurrently: number one, calmly direct Mom to look further for a button that says "Stop" or "Turn off Power;" number two, I could never have imagined being in the presence of my mother and a porn film at the same time; and number three, I wanted to get the hell out of here, NOW! And this third thought I shared with my mother on the spot.

"Neil," she said, "I hear you—I understand, and I have an idea. Let's just leave—walk out of here with the video still going."

And that's exactly what we did. We ran into no one as we slipped out of the office and walked back down the long hallway to the parking lot. As we swung onto the highway, my mother took my hand in hers and said, "Neil, I love you so much. No matter what, we will always be soul mates." She told me to put today behind me, that it wasn't important as long as she had me. She told me what a good sport I was and that she was so proud of the way I had, and still was, handling everything that had been thrown my way.

I nodded sadly, blinking back tears. I told her I loved her too, and I never felt it as strongly as that afternoon when we escaped together from the fertility clinic. We sat in silence for a spell. Maybe we were each suspended in our individual sadness at the way the day had played out. But then I heard her giggle.

"What," I asked.

"Nothing," she answered.

"I know what you're thinking, what little scenario you're imagining," I shot back.

"You think so?" she said.

"I know so," I answered back. "You're thinking of Maude wondering what's taking so long. Finally she hears the video end. She knocks on the door and when I don't answer, she comes in. And the only thing she finds is an empty, crushed-up collection cup for all her trouble."

"Yeah—that's about right," she admitted.

I didn't exactly give a belly laugh, but a half smile crossed my face.

ELEVEN

CHAMPION

Origin of the name "Neil"
Anglicized form of the Gaelic "Niall". It is believed to be from niadh (a champion); others think it is from niall (a cloud).
~ from babynamewizard.com

*a*NEWS OF NEIL'S STORY SPREAD. Because our goal was to resume as normal and natural a life as we could, we spent much time out and about, and Jim and I encouraged Neil to do so with as many different people as possible. He cut a dashing but very different kind of figure around town with his dark glasses, his white cane, and his muscled physique. He emanated an ease of well being. And, quite frankly, he was a curiosity. Seeing a blind person on town or city streets is fairly rare. I know. I am on the lookout for them wherever I go. And I admit to shamelessly bolting from conversations with friends in unfamiliar cities to run after a blind man or woman to introduce myself, to tell him or her that I have a blind son, to ask about their lives, to learn anything I can. I figure that, mostly, people like to talk about themselves, like to be noticed, like to be of help. I tell them they are helping me with my research. I am not shy in these situations because I am desperate to have it confirmed that people with a disability as profound as blindness can lead satisfying, fulfilling, normal lives.

Amazingly enough, after the harrowing experience speaking at the Greenwood School graduation, Neil developed a taste for public speaking.

Not long after his release from the hospital and rehab center, we had to deal with the issue of medical insurance. The Greenwood School's insurance benefits had been a godsend to Neil during his ordeal and we were grateful that he had been a full time employee prior to his medical emergency. Greenwood did everything possible to extend Neil's coverage for as long as possible, but we knew that we had to scramble to make other plans. Although Neil is now covered by a combination of Medicare and disability insurance through Greenwood, there was a gap before his current coverage could be instated. Hoops needed to be jumped through. Proof that he was permanently disabled took time to document and process. Luckily, we reside in the state of Vermont where health care for its children and low income citizens was being provided, at that time, through a coverage called Catamount. We applied, and Neil was accepted into the program.

Unfortunately, the United States economy began its descent into recession in 2008. Vermont was facing serious budget short-falls, and a solution proposed by then Governor Jim Douglas was to cut funding for health, education, and social programs which would disproportionately affect low income Vermonters, senior citizens, at-risk children, and the disabled. And, of course, it was rumored that the Catamount Insurance plan, which had been a model for other states, was on the short list for being cut or modified.

On a cold Monday night in the winter of 2008, Neil and I and his aunts Jane and Jean joined about fifty protesters holding white candles outside the Brattleboro Post Office. This gathering was one of ten Save our State vigils held throughout Vermont that evening and was organized by the Vermont Campaign for Health Care Security. The Brattleboro vigil had been organized by former nurse turned newspaper columnist and political activist, Richard Davis, who maintained that tax increases on higher incomes and an additional tax on cigarettes would provide needed revenues without undermining essential services and programs for citizens in need. At some point during the evening, the press came to take photos and interview some of the vigil participants. Richard introduced a reporter to Neil, and Neil ended up being interviewed and quoted in the newspaper the next morning.

As I stood beside Neil and heard him briefly recount his story to the reporter—how he had recently been employed at a full time job, had had to leave the position due to medical treatment as well as disability, how he was grateful and proud that he resided in a state that had cared enough about its citizens to provide affordable health care, and how he feared for himself and others if it should be cut—I noted how well he handled himself. He spoke with confidence and clarity. Later that evening, as he and his aunts and I sat in a downtown restaurant, we were in high spirits from our participation in the vigil and about Neil's role in providing a story and a voice for the public to connect to.

A couple of weeks later, during a week in which he was taking his chemo pills, Neil accompanied Richard Davis to the Vermont Statehouse in Montpelier in order to talk to the House Health Care Committee and tell them how proposed budget cuts would affect his life. Upon their return, Richard devoted his next weekly column to their experiences that day. An excerpt follows:

> Neil's testimony was passionate and articulate. A few of the committee members were in tears. He told his story and asked the legislators to think about what would happen to him if he could no longer afford his chemotherapy treatment.
>
> I explained to Neil how TV exposure would be compelling, and I got a newsman to bring his camera into the committee room to do a piece for the 6 p.m. news.
>
> While we were at the Statehouse, I introduced Neil to just about every legislator that had anything to do with health care reform. We also had a private meeting with Senate President Pro-tem Peter Shumlin who has known Neil for many years.
>
> It was a day of effective lobbying in the best sense. Neil lobbied on his own behalf and I tried to stay in the background as much as possible. My job was to be his guide dog, both politically and physically.

That Friday the 13th is a day I will remember
for the rest of my life. It was a day that both Neil
and I felt a tremendous surge of energy simply by
doing something that most people consider less
than honorable—lobbying. It was also a day that
revealed to me a 29-year-old man who will not let
a life-altering experience ruin his life. Despite an
uncertain future in a world of darkness, Neil has
managed to maintain a sense of humor about his
situation. He appreciated a bit of dark humor when
I introduced him to people as the Ted Kennedy
of Vermont, and we both had a little laugh when
his red and white cane tripped a legislator who
almost took a header onto the floor.

The four hours we spent in the car that day
changed my world. Even a nurse with thirty years
of experience still has a lot to learn. The image
of Neil getting lost in his house for the first few
months of his blindness haunts me. The ability
to joke with him about his blindness reminded
me that taking life too seriously can be an illness
without a cure...

The day in Montpelier was a life changing event for Neil
as well. Although health care reform did not become his area
of expertise or passionate cause, being the poster boy for the
disabled who live life to the fullest did.

~

Neil started being asked to speak to various groups. Some were comprised of individuals living with disabilities, some included students who were behaviorally challenged, some were regular junior high or high school classes whose teachers wanted to expose them to ways in which the disabled navigate the world in different ways. Neil and his friend Laura have been featured on local radio about their experiences in navigating downtown Brattleboro with a wheelchair and a white cane in an effort to initiate improvements for others with disabilities. During the year of coming to terms with his altered identity, Neil began to create a new self-identity, built from necessity. He had to make peace with the fact that the life he wanted was not to be. The life he got was all there was. Claiming it, embracing it, and living it to the fullest was the mission and adventure that lay before him.

~

Neil finished his twelfth and final round of chemotherapy in June of 2009. Results of his brain MRIs throughout the year had provided us with those happy trips home that put all of our other life problems in perspective. The year was over. We had done everything we could, but that very thought, the finality of it, made me jittery. Sitting with Dr. Renaud as he reviewed the MRI following our one year milestone, I asked him, outright, "So how has Neil done?"

He met my anxious gaze with an even, steady gaze of his own. "He's done very well. I'm pleased. I'm pleased with the results of the treatment, and I'm pleased with the way Neil is living his life. We'll see you in three months. If things continue as they are, we will extend check-ups to six months down the line."

As we exited the hospital and made our way down the sidewalk, Jim was on one side of me holding my hand, Neil on the other with his hand on my upper arm, his white cane making wide arcs in front of us. I don't think either of them noticed that I was walking on air.

～

Neil immediately started making plans for a celebration which he dubbed his "chemo-free" party. The day of the party was a perfect summer day. The swimming pool glistened, the grill sizzled, the sun radiated a warmth which was mirrored in everyone's heart for this day of happiness. It was a multi-generational party comprised of Neil's contemporaries, friends and neighbors who were Jim's and my contemporaries, even a few children, all gathered in love and support of Neil.

Just before the cake was brought out, Neil stood to thank everyone for coming. Much to the delight of the crowd, he had prepared little anecdotes about those who had played special roles in the year he had just lived through. It was a tribute to the angels who had surrounded him, upheld him, and offered him the greatest gifts—time, friendship, and the recognition that despite the monumental changes that had occurred, he was still Neil.

As I looked around at all the shining faces, I silently thanked them for their participation in our lives. The gathering that day was an affirmation that the full year was behind us. We had made it. The next chapter had not yet revealed itself, but I trusted that it would unfold and that Neil would be ready with the same optimism and courage that had carried him so far.

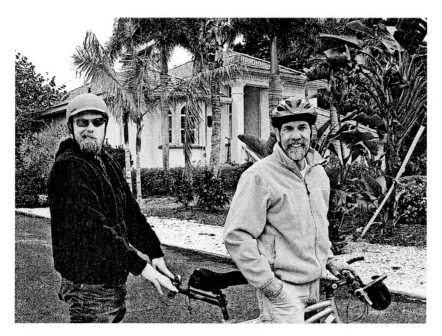

Above: Biking with Jim in Longboat Key, Florida

Below: Neil painting shelves in his new kitchen.

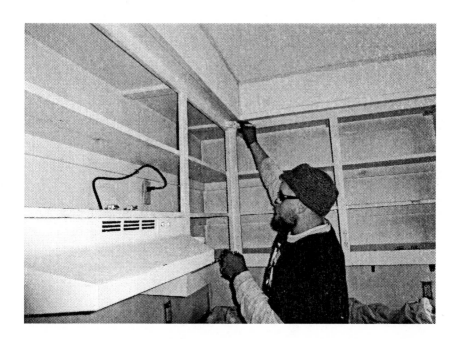

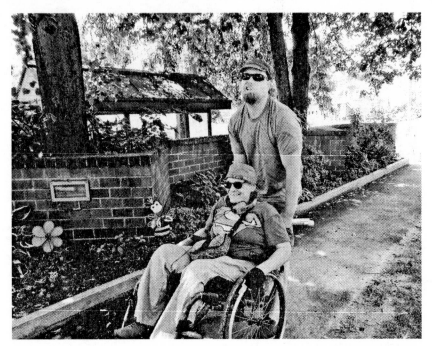

Above: Neil and Laura navigating their way through downtown Brattleboro, Vermont.

Below: The Blind Masseur, in residence and open for business.

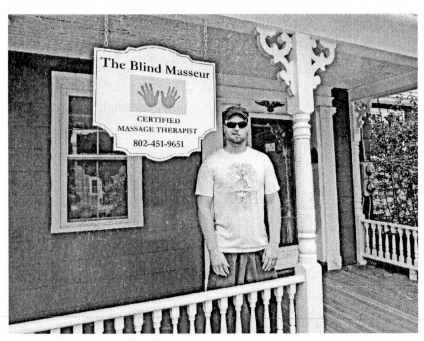

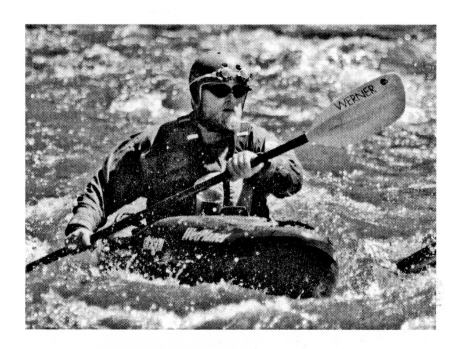

Above: Kayaking in Colorado with First Descents.

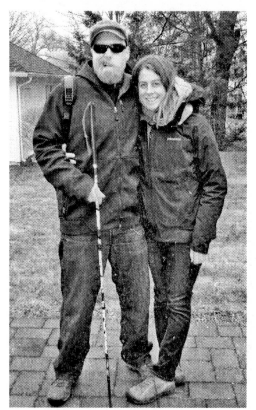

Left: Neil and Katy.

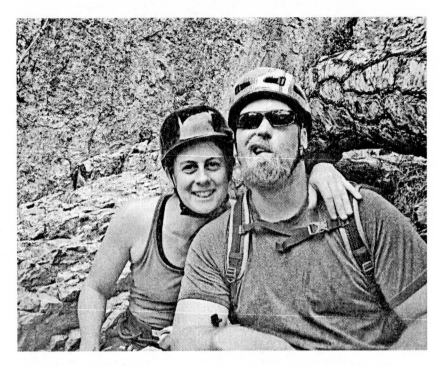

Above: Besides love for each other, Neil and Katy share a love of adventure and the outdoors.

Below: Neil climbing with Paradox Sports.

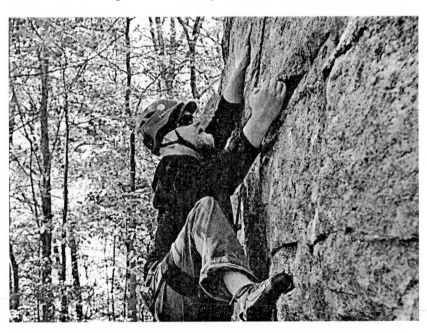

PART THREE

~

By Grit and by Grace

TWELVE

FLEDGLING

Whatever you can do, or dream you can, begin it,
Boldness has genius, power, and magic in it.

~ Goethe

*a*IN THE SUMMER OF 2009, NEIL informed us that he was planning to fly to Colorado to go white water kayaking with an organization called First Descents. I responded, "You're what?" I had no idea what he was talking about or where this crazy idea had come from.

He explained that Nick, his best friend from high school, had contacted him about the organization and had given his name and his story to the young founder, Brad Ludden, a world class, competitive white water rafter.

Brad had been deeply affected by his athletic aunt's journey with cancer. As Brad and his family supported his aunt through her treatment, he did some research. He learned that while considerable advances had been achieved in survival rates for both adults and children, the young adult population, from the teen years through the forties, had maintained very poor statistics in treatment efficacy and survival rates. Whether this was due to factors governing that stage of life or to the fact that much less cancer research had been devoted to this population had not been determined.

This knowledge affected Brad deeply. He, himself, was in that at-risk age group. He was an activist by nature, an idea man, and a believer in the body-mind connection. Using one's body, engaging in physical challenges, feeling success and pride in achievement all contribute to a sense of joy and well-being, independent of illness.

From these initial stirrings, combined with his enormous energy and drive, First Descents was born. Young adults living with cancer could choose to participate in one-week camps that featured either white water kayaking or rock climbing. The camps ran consecutively from spring to fall and were held in several of the western states. Aside from the athletic aspects of the camps, a campfire was held each night with sharing about the day's adventure, reflections on the nature of illness and well-being, healing rituals, tears and laughter. At the end of the week, participants returned home feeling uplifted and supported by new friends with whom they could genuinely open up—young people who were living life with similar fears and uncertainties.

First Descents had never had a blind participant. But Brad, being Brad, relished challenges and new opportunities. He decided, after speaking by phone with Neil several times, that Neil would be an ideal addition to the group. He envisioned an adaptation he felt would work with a blind athlete. At certain times, when it would be most helpful and/or necessary, he would kayak backward in front of Neil's kayak and give Neil verbal commands as to which way to aim and paddle.

Once Jim and I read a bit about First Descents, we were completely won over. We were thrilled that Neil would have the opportunity to once again experience himself as an athlete. And, of course, we knew that he would be a tremendous asset to any group in the social realm.

A vacation away from home for Neil was also a vacation for Jim and me. I feel no guilt in admitting it, as I realize that what we were truly getting was a respite from sorrow—the private agony of parents witnessing, on a daily basis, the struggles of their child whose life has taken a disappointing and irreversible turn and, for me, the exhaustion of always trying to make things right or, at least, better. Despite our unwavering love for one another, everyone needs some space and alone time. And both were scarce commodities the year Jim, Neil, and I lived under the same roof.

Neil called us often from Colorado. He was in high spirits from his adventures on the river and was moved by the activities at the evening campfires. He told us later that every day that week he witnessed the bravery, the resolve, the hope, and the inner strength of his fellow campers.

*n*THE PURPOSE OF FIRST DESCENTS is to give young people with cancer—and by young I mean people between the teen years and the late forties—an opportunity to get outside and do something challenging and fun, something they wouldn't normally do. The unique aspect is that the participants get to spend an entire week among others with similar life stories. Aside from the novelty of the climbing or kayaking experience, they are able to share the personal challenges they are living through.

As for me, I couldn't speak to anyone who was blind because I was the first blind participant in a First Descents program, but I could talk to young people who were dealing with life-threatening cancer. Some had just finished chemo, and some were actually doing chemo while they were at camp. Two or three participants, younger than I was, passed away not long after returning home from our week together. And that really shook me up. I remember their wonderful spirits. They were the nicest, kindest people, and it was hard for me to come to terms with their suffering and the fact that their lives ended at such a young age.

Regarding the campfires, I've always found this to be true: campfires, especially at night, open people up. Despite my blindness I can feel the physical heat, of course, but I can also sense the togetherness, the relaxation, and release that sitting around a fire instills in us. People relate to each other more deeply than they normally would.

Understanding this, First Descents designed various activities specifically for this evening ritual. One night we were all sent off to find two stones that appealed to us. On one we were asked to write a word that represented something we wanted to get rid of, something we wanted to expel from our life. Examples that people wrote were "fear," "pain," "grief," "anger." On the other stone we were asked to write a word that inspired us, like "courage," "resilience," "hope" or "love"—a word that symbolized a positive state of mind, one we hoped would be present as we lived our lives. We were given alone time to reflect on our stones with their competing sentiments, our positive and negative stones. Then we walked together to the river and were told to cast out the negative stone, to throw it out as hard as we could—skip it across the water. And the emotion that that stone held—just let it go. We were left with the stone that had the positive word and that one we were to keep. While in camp some of us kept our stones in our pockets, our backpacks, the breast pocket of our life jackets. Most of us planned to bring our affirmation stones home with us to put on a window sill or little altar Our stones were meant to serve as a powerful symbol, a concrete token of our aspiration.

Likewise, a tradition of First Descents was for all participants, campers and staff alike, to go by nicknames. I think the incentive for this was the positive aspect of leaving our daily identities behind, especially those identities that had been eroded by illness. Our new nicknames represented who we were outside of the stresses and fears of daily life—who we were at camp. We could think up our own nickname or get some help from others.

For me it was easy. I chose a nickname both my dad and I have used in our lives— "Tailz" from our last name Taylor. When I played lacrosse in college, my teammates called me Tailz. So that's my First Descents name. A fellow Vermonter was having a hard time coming up with a name for herself. When I found out she loved cheese I said, "Well, let's call you 'Cabot' after one of Vermont's brand name cheeses." She loved it and took it as her official nickname. There was Squirrel Girl, Chunky, Wildflower... you get the idea.

~

Prior to my cancer and blindness I had always loved adrenalin sports, and I knew that whitewater kayaking could be included in that category. I'd done a little kayaking on rapids when I was in high school— nothing serious. But I loved the videos I'd seen of guys going down the most ridiculous rapids ever. So when it came time to choose a First Descents program, I chose kayaking over the rock climbing camps. I'd always been comfortable in water, which, I learned, not all of the participants in the camp were. More power to them for showing up, being open to something scary, and taking a risk!

When my mom first heard of my intention to travel out west to go whitewater kayaking with First Descents, she assumed, at first, that I would participate in a tandem kayak. But that was never my intention. I was clear that I wanted my own kayak like everyone else. Obviously, my challenges were unique. It was scary hearing the rapids in the distance, perceiving their sound becoming louder and louder without being able to see what was coming up. But I began to become aware of the changing feeling of the water as the sound got louder. For the new me, using the combination of hearing and feeling allowed me to experience kayaking as an exciting adventure.

My biggest challenge was keeping the kayak straight as I went into a rapid. You never want to enter a rapid in a turned position, as this can cause the kayak to flip. Brad, as the most expert in rapids, became my leader. He had a bell on his kayak, and I would do my best to keep its sound directly in front of me.

If the bell sounded to my left or right, I'd readjust my kayak. We would do this to set up for the rapids, but once I was in the midst of them, I was unable to hear anything else. That's when I'd concentrate on feeling the rapids in my hips. I could feel which way the water was pulling, and I'd work my paddle. In whitewater kayaking, the paddle is paramount. It's what keeps you stable, and it must be kept in the water at all times.

These rapids, which seemed huge and challenging to all of us, were no big deal to Brad. And so sometimes when leading me he would go down the rapids backwards. Imagine that—huge swells—and he is paddling backwards! When we used the bell, navigating the rapids was all on me. When Brad paddled backwards, he could watch me and use his voice—"right-left-right-right." It was so much fun.

All kayakers can, and do, occasionally get caught in a swirl and flip over. And when this occurs, it happens in a flash. You can try to flip the kayak back to upright, but often you just have to eject. Whitewater kayaks are equipped with water-tight skirts, and when you eject you break that seal, but that's the way it goes. You and your kayak are now separated, but you never, ever abandon your paddle. When you come through a rapid, it's not as difficult to locate a kayak as it would a paddle. So when you eject, we were instructed to hang onto the paddle, get in a supine position, belly and feet up so as not to get caught on anything and sucked under, and just go with the experience until you emerge in quiet water.

When this happened to me, someone would grab my kayak, and I'd climb back in. Yeah, I ejected lots of times. The challenge is to not flip over, but when you do, well, that's fun too.

*a*NEIL RETURNED FROM HIS WEEK in Colorado with high spirits and greater confidence in himself. He was eager to continue moving ahead in his life. Upon his return I began to recognize a pattern in the fabric of our intertwined lives which was establishing itself as a sort of guiding rule. In order for the two of us to stay afloat, to keep plugging away in the face of a frightening illness and a catastrophic disability, we needed to immerse ourselves always in a plan with a next step and a goal to aim for. And Neil's new goal had become clear to him: to learn the skills he needed to live independently.

When I asked Neil recently when, exactly, the idea of attending The Carroll Center for the Blind and Visually Impaired was formed, he told me that he and Joe Stein had always thought an immersion program in independent living, offered in a residential setting, would be invaluable. Joe had sent other Vermont residents to the program and spoke highly of it. Neil was ready. He had completed his year of cancer treatment, was working out regularly, looked strong and healthy, and felt great. He was scheduled to move to the campus in Newton, Massachusetts, for a four month stay at the end of August 2009.

At the beginning of August, Neil, Jim, and I drove to Newton for an orientation that included about a dozen other individuals. The campus was compact but beautiful in the typical New England style: lush and green, venerable brick buildings intermixed with tasteful modern ones, and walkways, walkways, everywhere. In the case of The Carroll Center campus the walkways had not been constructed to keep students from ruining the manicured lawns or to add visual beauty to the setting. They were aids for blind students to walk independently from building to building by following them. To me, they seemed brilliant.

In contrast, the antique brick building that served as the residence hall where Neil would live during his time at Carroll seemed absolutely crazy to me. From the outside it was one of the quintessential ivy-covered beauties. Inside it was a maze of staircases and narrow corridors with bedrooms and bathrooms randomly placed at quirky angles. As we took the tour that late summer day, I thought to myself, "This would take ME some time to learn to navigate; it doesn't seem to be so user-friendly for the blind population!" But it wasn't an issue that Neil brought up during our frequent phone conversations over his first few weeks in residence. I came to think that perhaps the maze-like challenge was a good thing. It forced the residents to concentrate, to recall, to memorize, to practice orienting themselves in a space that mirrored challenges they would face in the wider world.

Following the campus tour that August day we gathered in a spacious room in one of the main buildings for the formal presentation by staff members. Looking around, I spotted a middle-aged man in the audience who was obviously blind. All the other participants seemed to enter the room and find seats without trouble. I figured that they were among the other category of students served by Carroll—the visually impaired. I remembered that Joe Stein had told us early on that total blindness is actually rather rare and that various scales have been developed to define both vision loss and blindness. Total blindness is the complete lack of form and visual light perception. Often, however, "blindness" is also used to describe severe visual impairment with some remaining vision. As of 2012 there were two hundred eighty-five million visually impaired people in the world of which two hundred forty-six million had low vision and thirty-nine million were blind.

I learned, as the orientation progressed that morning, that there was a room on the second floor, just above us, for the visually impaired to visit after the presentation. It featured displays of the newest aids designed to make independence at home and in the workplace easier to achieve for those with severely impaired vision. It was a stop on the tour we would not be making.

As the orientation continued, the familiar feeling of being overwhelmed and not capable of taking in everything around me began to set in. I know I was excited for Neil, but every next step carried an element of anxiety: would the program meet his expectations, would he be equal to the challenges, would there be too much free time and not enough activity to fill it? I took a few deep breaths. My head cleared and I relaxed into just being present for a new experience in a place I never dreamed I'd be.

A good deal of the presentation focused on technological advances that made being blind less challenging than it had been in the past. Some of the devises were described, some presented and briefly demonstrated. There was interest and a number of questions from the audience, many of whom were learning about these aids for the first time. I realized that some of the assembled that morning were living with progressive, irreversible vision loss. They did not yet need the support of these technological advances, but the day would likely come when they would.

And I realized how advanced, by necessity, Neil already was compared to most of the people in this particular group. He already owned and was comfortable using his Victor Stream Reader. The Victor held all his music, could be downloaded with audible books, could hold notes he wanted to record. While he still had much to learn in the area of computer skills, he was already using the program, JAWS, for voice activated e-mail, for typing text which was read back to him as he typed, and for downloading any information he wanted read to him. He had learned a great deal during the past year at home in Westminster West. Jim, always interested in technology, had done research about the best tools used by the blind community, and Joe Stein was a tremendous asset in accessing funds to ensure that Neil had what he needed. I squeezed Neil's hand, and he squeezed back. It was what I needed to confirm that he was feeling positive.

For me, the most meaningful aspect of the orientation that day, the part that I was hyper-alert to and will never forget, was being in the presence of three Carroll Center faculty members who were totally blind themselves.

Alex would have stood out in any crowd, not due to his blindness but due to his startling good looks. He was dark haired, dark complected, and beautifully dressed in a dark suit and tie. He had an air of quiet confidence and authority about him, and, indeed, he was one of the directors of the Center. He told us that he was filling in for the person who was scheduled to lead the orientation that day. Apparently, there had been a last minute change of plans, and he would, he said with a smile, do his best. He began speaking, and though I don't remember what he said, I noted how connected to him I felt. He was a skillful speaker, and I realized all of a sudden that although he couldn't see us, he acted as if he did. Unlike the blind speakers who followed him, he moved his head from the left side of the room to the right, in a way that made us feel noticed and included. He had mastered a powerful element of stage presence that eludes some sighted speakers. When he finished speaking, he said in an easy, offhand manner, "Now I'll take some questions. I am totally blind, so just call them out to me." Following the questions and answers, he thanked us for coming, urged us to visit all areas of the campus, and hoped we would enjoy the lunch that was being prepared for us.

I watched him turn to leave the podium. He turned left, his white cane in front of him. He headed toward the wall which would lead him, if he turned right and followed it, to the doorway at the back of the room. Against that wall, however, was a table, maybe always there, maybe there just today for the orientation. I watched as he bumped into it. His cane had probably arced the empty space below the table top. I didn't see it coming, that bump, but in an instant he simply turned and continued on his way toward the exit.

"So that's just the way it is," I thought. "It's not a big deal. Blind people are going to bump into things. And then they are going to reorient and continue on their way. And it's OK. It's not, necessarily, not supposed to happen. It happens." I craned my neck and watched that lovely man, with his beautiful posture and unscathed dignity, disappear through the doorway.

Peter, a technology teacher, addressed us next. He came down the aisle from which Alex had just left aided by one of Carroll's sighted employees who acted as his guide. They maneuvered in a way I had not seen before, most likely because the space was narrow. Peter walked directly behind his colleague with both of his hands on the other man's shoulders. They did, indeed, make a narrow footprint. Like Alex, Peter seemed completely unselfconscious with the method of mobility that worked best for him under the circumstances. He was there to address us, and that's what he got down to as soon as he reached the podium.

Peter's deportment in front of the group was more what you might expect from a blind individual. Unlike Alex he did not wear dark glasses, and, like most blind people, his eyes were unfocused. His gaze was straight ahead, which, until you became used to it, made you feel as though he was thinking out loud and unaware of being in the presence of an audience. Nevertheless, Peter impressed me by pulling a Victor Stream Reader and then an Olympus recorder from his jacket pockets and skillfully demonstrated how they worked. Everything he did was done by touch. Two words swirled in my mind as I gazed up at Peter standing before us—one was "serene," and I'll never know if, indeed he is, and the other was "capable," of which I have no doubt.

I don't recall the third blind presenter's name or area of expertise. But here is what I took away, and to me it was the most important and uplifting information of all because it was about his personal life: 1) he did all of his own banking on line; 2) he was married; and 3) his wife had given birth, just that week, to their second child.

His gift to me was this—"the world is full of possibilities beyond your imagination."

*n*I WOULDN'T SAY I WAS EXACTLY nervous about picking up and leaving what had once again become my home. I was more anxious to get on with it, to get the ball rolling in the area of my independence, to take the next step into my new life at this place Joe had described to me, The Carroll Center. My application had been accepted; I had attended an orientation, and now I was good to go—my next rehabilitation leap.

It's hard to say why the two weeks between orientation and my arrival for the Independent Living Program seemed like an eternity except that I was living in waiting mode. I was waiting for something I saw as monumental, something life-changing. I felt like a kid counting down to Christmas morning or my tenth birthday or summer vacation. At least the two weeks gave me plenty of time to pack my bag and consider the essentials I would need: the various drugs I took daily, my toothbrush, a stick of deodorant, several changes of underwear, and my Victor Reader which held my entire reggae collection—items I couldn't do without!

As I packed my bag, I tried to practice what I had already learned: to categorize and compartmentalize the location of every item. The first smallest pocket of my backpack held medicine and hygiene supplies, the next compartment, socks and underwear. Fortunately, at the time I was less of a clothes horse than I am today, so my attire did not require much room in my seemingly shrinking bag. I was aiming for efficiency. I didn't need to bring anything fancy. As I strained to zip up what I initially thought was a generous sized back pack, I mustered all the hope I could about my future prospects. My head swirled with wishful thinking about achievements that might lay ahead. I made a pact with myself to stay positive, no matter what I encountered, the hard parts along with the easily mastered.

When we finally arrived at The Carroll Center, we were warmly greeted by one of the directors and given a tour. I later learned that he had been blinded as a result of an injury he sustained during the war in Iraq. Somehow learning this helped put my malignant brain tumor in a new perspective. We suffer in different ways, but, in the end, we have to make the best of the hand we draw.

I was duly impressed by our guide's mobility skill as he led the way through the dorm to my room. As he ascended various staircases, punctuated by sharp turns and long hallways, he continued to talk, but my head was reeling with the effort of trying to make sense of the complicated-seeming route. The building reminded me of an impossible maze. Were they really expecting me to get around this convoluted place on my own? We finally reached our destination and entered a room on the right side of the hall—the room that was to be mine. I was overwhelmed. "But this is only day one," I told myself. "You gotta start somewhere, and I guess this here room will be my starting point."

It turned out that my roommate, Charlie, had arrived before me. I could hear him in the process of setting up his side of the room and noted that my side, closer to the doorway, would be easier for me to access and commit to memory. Whether this was purposeful on his part, I don't know, but I was grateful for this small break. I was heartened to discern immediately that Charlie, soon to be my new best friend, was outgoing and friendly. After a brief exchange he told us that he was going to the Common Room and quickly exited. I found out in short order that Charlie was not completely blind like me; rather, he had a degenerative disease that impaired his vision and, down the line, would take his sight altogether. The thought was chilling, and I couldn't decide which was worse, losing your vision overnight, like me, or slowly losing it day by day. I concluded that as terrible as it was, Charlie at least had some time to prepare for the loss.

After fifteen minutes of farewells and good lucks, my parents departed, leaving me alone in my unfamiliar new room. Remembering that I'd told myself that my room was my starting point in investigating the Carroll Center, I began to explore the space with my cane. I heard laughter down the hall, presumably from students who had been here for a while. While I didn't feel very lighthearted or even particularly social, I reminded myself that Charlie, a new resident too, was down there with the others, and I might as well follow his lead. I lay on my bed building up my courage. Finally, I got up and cautiously made my way out to the hallway. I headed toward the laughter on a mission to join my fellow dormmates.

∾

Although I am a social being by nature—I always longed for and sought out connections with others— here, in this unfamiliar, intimidating place, I found myself more reserved, more taciturn. At the beginning of my life at The Carroll Center I was more quiet than I'd ever been. Mostly I listened to the other students as they laughed and chatted, and I shared little of myself. I didn't have much in common, personally, with many of the residents. And I couldn't understand why they were so filled with exuberance during our free time in the Common Room. What were they so happy about? Were they not experiencing the same unfathomable loss that I was enduring?

What I came to realize after a few days was that over time they had bonded. And I could see that it was only natural that the newcomers, including the outgoing Charlie, would spend the first few days surveying the scene rather than diving right into the conversation. To top it off, I was out of practice meeting and associating with brand new people, and the idea of introducing myself or ingratiating myself with no visual cues was daunting. My life had taken such an abrupt turn. Nothing about it was the same as it had been. But I knew that I, too, had to change in order to adapt to the circumstances of this new life. So as awkward as it felt, I put myself out there in an effort to meet and connect with my fellow classmates. I never would have predicted it in those first few uncomfortable days, but by the third week I was assimilated into the crew of the visually impaired and newly blind. I felt halfway at home. I guess this is how it works at The Carroll Center surrounded by people on the same boat as you. Despite it being a depressing cruise liner, you are all passengers together.

Unlike my roommate, there were others at Carroll who were dealing with the shock of becoming blind very suddenly. A few individuals had lost their sight due to traumatic head injuries; one woman I became friends with had suffered the same fate as me after being diagnosed with a malignant brain tumor. I was surrounded by people I never would have met outside the Center, let alone become close with. I came to appreciate the fact that I bonded with such an eclectic group of people, people from different locations, ethnicities, races, ages, gender, sexuality, and socioeconomic backgrounds. Some had PhDs from prestigious universities, and others had not earned high school diplomas. All of these differences, which might be so front and center in the outside world, seemed microscopic compared to what we all had in common. Blindness does not discriminate in the same way that we human beings regrettably do. Everyone at The Carroll Center was present for the same reason: to learn how to live life without the benefit of sight. Before my arrival I had never even met a fellow blind individual, and here I was surrounded by them. Somehow it made me feel more "real," more validated as a human being who would make it through life, dark glasses, white cane and all.

~

Without a doubt, the most essential training at Carroll was mobility training. The whole campus, inside and outside, was the venue, the laboratory, the classroom, for the study and practice of how to navigate in the world. Luckily, I got the pick of the litter when it came to mobility instructors. Naomi and I hit it off right away, mainly because we had similar senses of humor. We were not afraid to laugh at ourselves (or maybe just at me!). She knew what a formidable task it was trying to get around both the inside and outside of the campus. I teased her that I'd come to believe I was in the middle of a cruel prank against the newly blind. I imagined, especially in the dorm building, a circus-type maze of mirrors. You turn the corner sure of where you are, only to run into another strategically placed mirror designed to mess with your head. She chuckled and assured me that eventually I would learn the lay of the land.

We started out using my small recording device so I could access my own verbal directions when I was on my own. We recorded directions to every building and classroom I needed to get to. We started with the most basic—the route from my room to the bathroom. And this is how it sounded: "Exit room and take immediate right. Track down this right wall 'till after several paces the hallway takes another right. Keep tracking the new hallway until you locate the first door, also, conveniently, on the right. That's the bathroom." Naomi reminded me that it would not be difficult to return to my starting point. Now all the rights were lefts, and the order was reversed.

It sounds simple, but for me it wasn't. It gave me a headache. I joked that I had been a math teacher prior to my blindness, and now I couldn't even keep track of the number of paces I was attempting to count! My sense of direction had been sketchy even when I was sighted. Now this weakness was more front and center than ever, affecting my progress. But I practiced this same bedroom to bathroom and back again route over and over until it was branded into my brain. I was convinced that if those on the outside world could witness my practice treks, they'd be convinced that I was a crazy person with a bent toward fumbling repetition. But Naomi was right. Despite my initial doubts, navigating the interior of the dorm eventually became second nature to me.

She also started, on day one, orienting me around the campus grounds. First we practiced navigating from one building to the next by relying on the handrails; then I used my cane to probe for the purposely placed landmarks which took the place of railings in some areas. Because I felt it would be a real faux pas to show up late for my classes or mealtimes, I began practicing these routes over and over on my own, as I had in the dorm. In the beginning, I needed to be rescued at least once a day by one or another of the panic-stricken faculty as they caught me way off course, headed confidently toward a busy thoroughfare. They were, nonetheless, ever supportive of my independent efforts, and we developed a familiar, friendly rapport. Eventually, even on the outdoor campus, I became more adept, and with it came some pride in my growing accomplishment.

~

Even after becoming blind, I found the most joy in physical endeavors— anything that might reawaken the athlete I had always been and that was now hibernating deep inside me longing to find an outlet. Surprisingly, an outlet was waiting at The Carroll Center in a form that was totally unfamiliar to me. One of the classes on my schedule was fencing. When I learned that I was to participate in this class twice a week, I was not immediately very enthusiastic. How are blind people supposed to sword fight? But other than mobility training, it was the only physical endeavor offered. I decided, despite my preconceived notion that it was a "fringe" sport, to start the class with the optimism I had promised to bring to everything during my time at Carroll.

Apparently Ramon, the instructor, was renowned in the small world of fencing. He was fully sighted and openly enthusiastic about teaching his passion to a small group of blind individuals. During the first class, two other students and I were introduced to the equipment we would be using. First, of course, was the foil which we were encouraged to examine with our hands. Ramon made it clear that if we mistakenly called it a sword, we'd owe him twenty push-ups, no debate. I worked my hands up and down its length. The thin foil was about three feet long and, unlike a rigid sword, it was quite flexible. The business end of the foil had a metal tip; the other end sported a handle, designed to protect your hand, with a mysterious cord extending from its base. The cord was attached to a box which would expel a resounding beep when a successful strike compressed the tip of the aggressor's foil. The rest of the gear consisted of a well-padded long sleeved jacket and a face protector, which, in my imagination, looked like an item from a science fiction or fantasy book. The front was made of thick metal mesh. It was designed to protect the face while at the same time (our group excluded) offer a full view of an opponent. When the mask was pulled down, it fully encompassed the head, rendering the fencer unidentifiable. Whenever I pulled that mask down, I felt strangely empowered. It brought me back to the memorable fencing scene in the classic film *The Princess Bride* in which I had, in my youthful imagination, starred as the hero. Now, here I was, years later, blind, but holding a foil in my own hand.

What most people probably don't realize about fencing is that it all takes place on a one dimensional level. Unlike movie scenes where the duel takes the participants all around the set, jumping from rocks and swinging across crevasses, fencing is a straight-on encounter. There is no stepping aside to avoid a blow. Instead, you use your foil to parry your opponent's thrust or step back in a defensive move. This makes it much easier for blind fencers because the motion of the body is simply front or back. You don't go around your opponent but straight through him! The three of us in the class took turns fencing with each other. The memory of the sound of our metal foils clanging as they connected still gives me a slight rush of adrenaline. I came to the conclusion that fencing was a more graceful (not to mention non-violent) form of sword fighting which required as much, if not more, finesse.

Of course, without sounding pompous, I excelled at it and

couldn't get enough! If I had a free period I would go see if I could participate in another class. Luckily Ramon indulged me by suiting up himself then defeating me in short order. I never got a single successful strike on him, but it never mattered to me. He made me realize that despite being blind I could still experience enjoyment in a new athletic endeavor. While for me it would never be fencing that I'd ultimately pursue—I mean how many of your friends have weekend fencing parties?— he planted the seed inside me that there were other physical endeavors out there that I could learn to enjoy despite my limitations. It was up to me to go out there and find them.

~

Not all of the classes at Carroll were totally out of the realm of my prior experience. But who would have thought that woodworking with power tools could be adapted for the blind? My dad had been a carpenter even before I was born. He had built our first house with my mother as his sole assistant and had been a building contractor for most of my younger years. So I was familiar with and took a liking to constructing things with my own hands.

Those were the happy, confident thoughts on my mind as I descended the long staircase that led to the woodworking shop. As I entered, another class was about to end. This class had been at Carroll for a while, so they were experienced and seemingly at home in the shop. At least this was my impression, as I could barely hear the instructor walk toward me and greet me amid the cacophony of power tools the students were using.

Ron welcomed me with an enthusiastic handshake, and I noted that his hand was strong and heavily callused. The veteran class shut down their tools and departed, with farewells to Ron. Suddenly the room seemed eerily quiet, and the feeling that welled up in me was not what I had expected. Here I was on Day One of the class, a class that I felt some affinity for, and suddenly I didn't even want to be in the same room with a table saw. Forget that I initially thought I'd be a competent student and maybe a bit ahead of the game due to my background. Now I could only conjure up the image of a dismembered finger spurting blood all over the workshop. Nonetheless, I was signed up for this class, and I told myself that I would adjust as I had in so many other arenas.

My saving graces were that we did not start using the power tools right away—a total relief— and that the class was so small that if it weren't being held in a fully equipped woodworking shop, I would call it intimate. There were only three of us, enabling Ron to give us the individual attention we all needed. Ron proved to be not only an expert in the area of woodworking but an expert working with and relating to blind people. He was a genuinely nice guy with a never-ending supply of bad jokes to lighten the mood and entertain us.

We began our study working with small finger puzzles designed to support and strengthen our fine motor skills and our perception. The puzzles required us to insert little wooden pins into holes that were scattered on a four by four inch board and "feel" how to create a shape— first a triangle and then increasingly more complicated figures that Ron directed us to build. This was very challenging and, as in so many endeavors, made me realize how we humans rely on our visual sense first and foremost for success in almost all situations. An additional difficulty for me was that my weaker hand continued to hamper my dexterity. I could have sworn that the pins were all too large to fit into any of the minuscule holes. It frustrated me to the point where I wanted to throw the stupid little puzzle across the room. But, once again, The Carroll Center instilled in me a valuable life lesson: a task that seems utterly impossible at first is often achieved with patience, perseverance, and an openness to thinking in new, more expansive ways.

To me, this class was such a special part of the curriculum because it emphasized the value and the power of our sense of touch. Our tactile sense, in some cases, can substitute for the eyes. Obviously, hands cannot provide the splendor of a beautiful sunrise, but they can send enough information to your brain to implement tasks and projects you never thought were possible.

We learned to use rulers with tactile marks that signified every measurement up to an eighth of an inch. After some practice, I became proficient at measuring using this new method. Similar to a pencil in the hands of a sighted person, I used a metal tipped utensil which left a slight indentation on the wood, showing me where to align my saw for a cut.

It took a good two weeks for me to let down my guard in the presence of the menacing sound of the power saws. Probably because I'd relied on vision to assess danger my whole life, sounds now seemed amplified. My fear in the woodworking shop was nearly identical to my fear of the sound of traffic bearing down on me even when I knew I was safe on the sidewalk. In both cases I felt completely exposed to bodily danger. And here in the shop, my fear was very specific—the absolute vulnerability of my fingers.

Our first step in learning to use the saws was simply to turn them on!—to be up close and personal with the feel, the sound, and the mechanics of their properties and use. We then progressed to practicing the simple act of cutting a piece of scrap wood. These were the baby steps, and we all appreciated this simple sequence. Ron's carefully crafted tutelage was just what I needed to help me overcome my initial fear. He always emphasized taking our time, even after we had progressed to cutting a required length which we had carefully measured and marked. He always told us there is no race in using the saw: don't even consider making a cut until you feel very sure. And to be on the safe side, be conservative. You can make as many cuts as necessary to adjust for not quite meeting the mark the first time. One of our mottoes became, "You can take a little off, but you can't add it on."

Halfway through the course we were required to come up with an individual project, ideally something we could use in our personal lives. My idea, which then became my plan, was to build a shoe rack for the apartment I hoped I would move into following my stay at Carroll. In my old life, my shoes lived in a haphazard pile near the door. My new life as an increasingly independent blind person called for something different, something that would support my need for a more orderly and organized existence.

Using all the methods Ron had taught me, making careful measurements, using my fingers to substitute for my eyes, I began to construct the shoe rack that I had designed in my mind's eye. In the process, I must have made a hundred cuts with the table saw, realigning the blade again and again. Due to my fastidiousness I never made a cut too short. After nearly a month, with the precision of a surgeon, I completed the project. I was so proud of the shoe rack and, adding to my elation, Ron seemed just as proud. He put it on display during my last weekend at Carroll so families could see the impressive projects coming out of the Center's woodworking department. He asked if he could snap a few photos of it for his scrapbook. I assured him that not only did I not mind, I would be honored to have my shoe rack memorialized in the archives of The Carroll Center. The shoe rack sits in the entryway of my home to this day.

Shortly before my graduation from The Independent Living Program, I completed a live-alone simulation which every graduate must undergo. Using all the practical knowledge I'd gained from the classes in life skills, I moved from the dorm to a small on-campus apartment for three days and two nights. Now, instead of showing up for the hearty meals I'd come to look forward to and always overindulged in at the dining hall, I was not welcome there. I was expected to cook all of my own meals and spend a good deal of time on my own.

My cooking teacher and I made a trip to the supermarket with a carefully crafted list and a mere fifty dollars. The way I was eating then—indulging in the endless supply of egg and sausage sandwiches every morning and the sweet finale of ice cream sandwiches after dinner— this budget would barely cover breakfast! But I was excited nonetheless. Given the fact that I had been practicing for this final exam for the past three months, I ended up passing with flying colors. However, my skills faltered a bit (and were noted in my final assessment) when it came to cleaning up after my effusive cooking efforts.

Things "escaped" me as they probably do for all novice blind cooks. Whether it was a remnant of chicken, an errant slice of pepper, or a fragment of egg shell, I left my mark. But the fact that my final score dipped a bit in the hygiene and tidiness department did not negate the truth that I had learned to make a finger-lickin' good chicken stir fry. And if you had been my guest for dinner during my solo you would have had to lick your fingers, as I elected not to buy napkins with my meager allowance. I know when the apartment was reviewed after my stay, there were a few spots that my sponge had missed, but I joked with my instructor that I blame it more on my innate messiness than my lack of sight. I wish, I told her, that she could have viewed my stove top when I was fully sighted. If she had, I'm sure she would have decided to dramatically elevate my final score!

At the end of my three day stay in the test apartment, I was completely comfortable and a little sad to leave the peaceful serenity of my personal space. As I packed my bag to move back into the dorm, however, I realized how eager I was to re-enter the social scene of what now felt like "my people." My assimilation took a good five minutes of slapping hands with my visually impaired buddies and getting welcome home hugs from my blind and visually impaired lady friends. I fell right back into the relaxation of being with my "peeps," laughing and bantering the evening away while lounging around on the big couches in the common room. Now and then it would cross my mind that I might like living in this blind-friendly world forever. But the thought would fade almost as quickly as it had formed. The stronger, more rational part of my consciousness knew that this microcosm was temporary and was designed to prepare me for my assimilation back into the real world.

*a*NEIL WAS HOME FOR FOUR DAYS over Thanksgiving. He would return to Carroll for three more weeks and then return to Vermont just before Christmas at the conclusion of his program. He announced that he was ready to find an apartment and fulfill his goal of living independently.

Neil's friend George had sold his home in Westminster West and moved into a spacious brick apartment building called the Manly Building in downtown Brattleboro. He had been in touch with Neil and had let him know that a tenant in the building was moving out and that the vacated apartment would likely be available to rent following some renovations. He was ready to put in a good word about Neil to the landlords. Neil was excited. He had already made the decision to move to Brattleboro where he would be within walking distance of restaurants, the food coop, a downtown drug store, and his bank. He would be centrally located, enabling friends to easily drop by. Rural settings in which Neil had resided for most of his life no longer suited his circumstances. He was eager for new surroundings to support his new life.

Neil placed a call and left a message with the agency that managed George's apartment building. We also perused the "for rent" section of the newspaper to explore other possibilities in the downtown area, and he left his name and number for an apartment listed just across the street from George's building. By the time he needed to leave again for The Carroll Center, his calls had not been returned, and he was disappointed. I told him, "Neil, absolutely nobody does business over a major holiday like Thanksgiving. I'm not surprised that you haven't received a call. But there's no reason to think that you won't."

He agreed but felt at loose ends. "I'll be out of state, and I don't want to risk losing one of these apartments. And they're located in the area I most want to be," he answered. "Would you and Dad be willing to go check them out? I would need you to go with me anyway, and you can judge if either of them would be a good place for me to live."

The next week a call came in from the co-owner of George's building. I told her that Neil would be out-of-state for the next three weeks, was eager to relocate to Brattleboro, and had given his dad and me permission to view apartments in his behalf. We agreed to meet the following day. Jim took the call for the second apartment and scheduled a viewing for the day after our first appointment. I couldn't believe this was happening! Neil was actually going to be moving into a place of his own, starting a new chapter. I was excited for him and ever so proud of how far he had come. And then, because I'm me, a worry niggled in. It was one I had to think on, needed advice about, so I called Joe Stein at his office.

"Joe," I confided, "I'm calling because I'm worried. Neil's asked us to check out an apartment tomorrow in Brattleboro. Jim and I are meeting the owner at four o'clock. I didn't say anything to her about Neil on the phone. I don't know if she knows that Neil is blind or not. She might, because his good friend lives in the building and may have mentioned that Neil would be contacting her. But what if she decides that she doesn't want to rent to a blind person? What if she thinks it's too great a risk? What if she thinks he'll leave a burner on and start a fire?" I had gotten myself really worked up.

Joe listened to me in his usual calm and patient manner. "Well, I don't think you should be too worried," he said. "I don't think it will be an issue. If you feel that it is, have her call me." I hung up feeling relieved. How lucky we were for Joe's continued role in our lives!

The following afternoon, as Jim and I pulled alongside the solid brick building that housed Neil's potential apartment, we noted immediately how accessible the front door was to the adjacent public parking lot. This is where we would park when we came to visit Neil or pick him up. Yes, we would have to put money in the meters, but we would never have to drive around looking for a spot to park. Although we'd never really paid attention to this apartment building before, we had walked past it countless times. It's first floor housed a gift shop, a small store-front skin care and massage studio and a popular restaurant where I could picture Neil and friends meeting for breakfast from time to time. We met the owner in the hallway as we ascended the short stairway that led to the second floor.

"You must be the Taylors," she greeted us with a warm smile. "I'm Joanne." She immediately put me at ease. "The apartment is right at the end of this hall."

We turned and gazed down the wide, old-fashioned corridor. "What could be better," I thought as we followed her, "than Neil's apartment being at the very end of the hallway—no counting doors on a side wall. He'll know he's home when his cane hits the far wall: the end of the line."

She unlocked the door and led us into an expansive, unfurnished living room. At the end of the room, facing us as we walked through the door, was a bank of windows that overlooked Mt. Wantastiquet which presides over Brattleboro's downtown. Although Neil could never experience the visual pleasure of having our landmark mountain framed in his living room windows, I knew he would love knowing it was there. Anyone else entering the apartment would be enchanted by the unexpected view. The room was a blank slate waiting for a new owner who would design an arrangement that would work for him and the friends who spend time with him.

The kitchen, to the right, was large and homey like a farmhouse kitchen of the past. It had plenty of tall wooden cupboards, ample counter space, and room for a table and chairs by the windows which overlooked High Street. The same living room wall that led to the kitchen had another doorway just beyond the kitchen's entrance. It opened onto a short, narrow hallway, narrow enough for a guy Neil's size to stretch out both arms and touch the walls on each side for orientation. To the left was the bathroom and at the end was a cozy square bedroom, also overlooking High Street.

The apartment couldn't have been more straightforward. Memorizing new interior spaces was still fairly new for Neil, but I felt that this apartment lent itself to a beginner. I fell in love with it at once, imagining that if I were a single person looking for an apartment, I would take this one immediately. I looked at Jim and could see that he, too, was impressed. I knew our family would feel at home in this space. I hoped it was just waiting for Neil!

Jim asked Joanne if she was aware that Neil was blind. She knew it already and was happy to welcome him to the building. I breathed a sigh of relief and gratitude. We told her that we loved the apartment, that Neil was planning on phoning us that night for our impressions, and could we let her know in the morning if we were a definite "yes"? The plan was fine with her.

When Neil phoned us that evening, I was bursting. "Neil!" I gushed, "Dad and I saw the most perfect apartment this afternoon. We loved it, and I'm positive that you'd love it too!"

"No way!" he shouted. He was laughing and whooping at the same time. I described the layout to him in as much detail as I could, hoping he could form an adequate picture in his mind.

"What do you think?" I finished. "Do you feel like you can make a decision about it, or would you rather wait until you can be here in person?"

"Call Joanne in the morning," he responded without hesitation. "Tell her the deposit check's in the mail, and I can't wait to move in. And thank you guys so much!"

I relayed Neil's message to Joanne the next morning. Jim left a message with the managing agent of the apartment building across the street: "Please cancel our appointment to see the apartment for rent. We've made other plans."

n IT'S TRUE I HAD BEEN DISCOURAGED in my first attempts at making contact with landlords of downtown apartment buildings that may have been suitable for me. And I returned to Carroll feeling that this next stage might not move ahead as expected. In all honesty, I guess that although I knew the upcoming goal was to live on my own in my own space, I just couldn't actually imagine it happening. No matter how hard I tried not to be, and despite continuously trying to convince myself of my own competence, I was anxious when I thought about living alone. But the funny and, I guess, positive spin was this: though I couldn't rid myself of the vague doubts that would come and go, usually when I was lying in bed after a long day, I was equally excited about the whole idea and could recognize and believe in all the progress I had made here at Carroll.

My mother called after dinner one evening, and from the

excitement in her voice I could tell that my confidence issues in no way had been transferred to her. In her mind I was "good to go." Not only was I glad I had covered myself successfully in front of my family, but her confidence served to bolster my own. She told me that she and Dad had gone to view the apartment in the building where George now lived—the best location in town—not directly on but perpendicular to Main Street.

She described the cozy entrance where we could fit a chair, a great place to sit and kick my boots off before hanging my jacket on the facing wall. She led me into a generous, light-filled living room with a space to the left that could accommodate an elliptical running machine. She instructed me to think "right-hand turn from the entrance" where I'd enter a kitchen with a long expanse of counter that ended in an empty space under a window where a table was meant to be. She described the positions and layout of the bathroom and bedroom. I tried to see the whole apartment with Mom as my verbal sighted guide. It sounded perfect in every way. How could I say no? It seemed that my parents had just seen the place that was to be my new home, and there was no point in looking further. We had lucked out on the very first appointment.

As I lay in bed that night I kept thinking about my apartment. I already thought of it as mine. I managed to suppress the slight anxiety I felt about leaving the blind amenities of the Carroll Center behind and setting off to live on my own by repeatedly reviewing the blueprint Mom had provided. I was in bed in Newton, Massachusetts, but in my mind I was miles away in a town that I'd soon call home. I had to laugh at myself. How different these bedtime musings were from those of my younger, wilder, sighted days. Back then my fantasies took the form of me on an important mission, often fueled by themes of the video games I played. Now, instead of protecting planet Earth from evil, invading aliens, I was on an equally challenging mission of making it from my imaginary bedroom to my imaginary bathroom in my imaginary apartment because I was desperate to take a pee!

Of course I realized that my internal map of my soon-to-be new digs was most likely upside down and backwards. It probably would have been for anyone, sighted or blind. I needed the chance to check out the real place—work it over with the swooping back and forth motion of my new sense organ, my ever-present white cane, accompanied by its twin tool, my extended left arm. Between these two new tactile accommodations and what one of my friends has come to call my "one armed zombie on heavy barbiturates" walk, I would start to memorize my new home. But at the present moment, in my head, I was a perfectly coordinated traveler, and until the time came, the mental map I had crafted would have to suffice.

*a*SHORTLY BEFORE NEIL'S GRADUATION FROM The Carroll Center Jim's brother Tom, an inveterate tag sale aficionado, known for his often outlandish purchases, came upon a stack of four Playboy magazines on a table in someone's yard—all in braille. They were very thick, the color of brown paper shopping bags, had the Playboy bunny logo displayed prominently on the cover and had, obviously, no photos. He purchased them at once and brought them to Vermont at Christmas time. We roared with laughter when he pulled them out of the bag, placed them on Neil's lap, and told him what they were.

Neil let out a war whoop: "Tommy—you are the man! These are so cool! I can't wait to show them to all my friends!"

Tom asked, "Can you make any sense of the braille? Can you read any of it?"

Neil answered, "Not really, but I have a great use for them!"

Jim and I didn't realize at the time of this humorous gift that as part of the Carroll ceremony, each graduate is asked to give a short speech. On the afternoon of Neil's speech, which Jim and I listened to later on tape, Neil talked about how grateful he was that The Carroll Center was there for him when he so desperately needed it. He thanked Joe Stein and the state of Vermont for making his stay possible financially. He told the assembled crowd that he'd learned to make a mean pan of scrambled eggs under Marjorie's tutelage, that he'd gained confidence in his mobility skills with the guidance and unwavering encouragement of Naomi, that he couldn't wait to use the shoe rack he'd made with Ron in the woodwork shop, that the time he'd spent learning to fence had greatly helped his balance, that the computer training had given him the foundation he needed to move forward and increase his skills each day.

"All of this training will help support me as I move toward my goal of becoming as independent as I possibly can be." He paused.

"Oh! One more thing. I totally forgot to thank my braille

instructor for his patience as I attempted to learn more of the basics of braille. To show my gratitude, I wanted to leave a little gift for The Carroll Center library to inspire future braille students."

Apparently, he raised both hands high above his head and the audience of staff and students—at least the ones who could see—gazed up at two of the giant braille Playboys. The crowd went wild. Hooting, laughter, and clapping filled the room as the seeing audience described the scene to the blind and visually impaired. As he was being assisted to his seat, Neil remembered to call out to the crowd, "Of course I just bought these for the articles!"

THE DAY FOLLOWING MY GRADUATION, when I bequeathed to the school a portion of my braille Playboy magazines amid a raucous crowd, my family arrived to pick me up. After half an hour of tearful good-byes, congratulations, and let's-keep-in-touch phone number and e-mail exchanges, my Carroll Center days were behind me. My parents and I made our way toward the Vermont border, and all the while I shared my experiences of everything I had done and learned over the past several months. If I felt nostalgia at the time, I don't recall it, because foremost in my radar was the new apartment that was waiting for me. But I did have the sense that I was straddling two worlds.

It was just before Christmas, and I had paid rent for the last two weeks of December in order to furnish and arrange my new home while my brother and sister were home for the holidays. I would officially be in residence by the first of January, which seemed like an appropriate time to start anew. In the meantime, it felt good to be returning to my family home where the five of us could spend time together like we had every other Christmas.

I had moved into a reflective mind state after all my enthusiastic sharing when my father announced, "What the heck— let's get off the highway at Exit Two and check out the Manley Building!" We all got into a kidding mood about the name of my new building—how we chose the apartment in order to elevate my status in the world. We parked in the lot which abutted the left side of the building and made our way to the front door. And I got to experience for the first time the straightforwardness of locating my own apartment from the street-side entrance. Of course it would take more than a few days of practice to "get it" on my own, but there were not that many complicated sequences or steps to memorize, and I felt confident I could master it in fairly short order.

As we stood in the hallway before my own door, I heard Dad pull out his key ring, and as he fumbled for the right key, I was more than champing at the bit. I think I practically pushed him out of the way in anticipation of entering and familiarizing myself with my future home. I wanted to feel out every aspect of the space—walk the footprint I'd been imagining since my mother's description.

I could sense the largeness of the living room immediately, could feel its emptiness, awaiting the furniture that would make it my own. I saw, in my mind's eye, the view of Mount Wantastiquet from the bank of living room windows. I tracked two walls and found the doorway to the kitchen where I ran my hands down the length of Formica. In both the living room and the kitchen I guided myself around the perimeters, and my mother walked me into the center of each room. I headed down the narrow hallway to the bedroom and bathroom by myself, exploring each space in my own way. I couldn't stop from grinning. This apartment was mine, and I was so proud of it already. Could things get any better? I wanted to compliment my mother; all the elements she had described, including the position of rooms, were pretty much as I'd pictured them

I made my way back to the living room where my parents were quietly talking. Mom broke off her conversation with Dad to ask me the question that, at this point, we all knew the answer to, but still she asked it: "Neil, what do you think? Can you picture yourself living here?"

I could feel my emotions overtaking me as I answered her in a voice three octaves above my normal pitch. "I love it: thank you for being such wonderful scouts!"

My dad spoke up then, probably to ward off the awkward sob-fest he saw coming on. "Neil, you did a fairly good job of checking out the place, but I notice you favor your right side so you missed a key element of the apartment."

I would have begged to differ with him, defending my highly improved caning skills, but this was the same observation pointed out to me again and again by my teachers at Carroll. So without putting up a protest, I guided myself back to the front door where I spun around and reset myself for another investigation. This time I would not miss anything.

I headed left from the entryway and again entered the living room. I swung my cane, and it immediately collided with what felt like a formidable object. I swiped my right hand through the air until it made contact with what felt like a metal cylinder. I grasped the cylinder and slowly slid my hand across it until the metal ended in a rubber encasement. I recognized that this was some sort of handle. I put some pressure on it with my arm and the handle pushed away in a familiar, perfectly aligned arc. I knew exactly what it was!

Before my mother could blurt out any precautionary words, I performed one of the only actions that was still automatic and that I was well trained to do. Using the rubber handle I gracefully (not an adjective I can use much anymore to describe my physical endeavors) pulled my feet up onto what I knew would be the foot pads, and I was off and running at an easy pace on my brand new elliptical runner!

I shouted out a holler of joy as my parents laughed and clapped. I dismounted, slightly out of breath, partly because of my unexpected physical exertion and partly because of the excitement of it all. I gave my father a bear hug, pretending to pick him up. I was overwhelmed with happiness as we collected our gear and locked the door behind us. And then he handed me the keys!

The next week was a week of merriment for me. I was reunited with my family, sharing stories of my experiences at The

Carroll Center and dropping in at my new apartment to plan the layout once the furniture was lugged in. My brother and sister were as impressed with my new home as my parents and I had been. Jessica was a natural at seeing the place through my sightless eyes and at planning the accommodations that would make the space highly functional and user friendly. Jackson jokingly suggested that I hang a basketball hoop in the living room. In their own ways they brought light into my world that week while the apartment brought a whole new sense of pride into my being.

But even more than that, I was proud of my family and their adjustment to the son and brother I had become and was still becoming, and of myself, for coming so far in building the competency to live on my own—something that once sounded like nothing but a fairy tale.

THIRTEEN

ASCENT

*Tell me
What is it you plan to do
with your one
wild and precious life?*

~ Mary Oliver

*n*LIVING IN THE HEART OF BRATTLEBORO was refreshingly different from living in rural Westminster West where I'd spent my first year of blindness. There was so much going on right outside my door! In-town living erased many of the transportation problems that the blind have to deal with daily. I took an Introduction to Insight Meditation class in hopes of finding some inner peace. While my mother drove me to the first class, almost immediately my fellow classmates, many of whom lived in town, eagerly volunteered to take turns picking me up. It was not a hardship for them as my apartment was so easy to swing by. I went way out on a limb, taking a dance class with my friend Amelia at a local studio. It was only a short stint: after disrupting the whole class by crashing into an assortment of tables and chairs while trying to learn the Lindy Hop, I eventually hung up my dancing shoes. But I didn't let it dampen my spirits. The point is, I could try out and participate in nearly anything I cared to.

The Manly Building became a small but supportive social network for me. Now I had neighbors in close proximity—really friendly people who were more than willing to help me assimilate to my new environment. We could knock on each other's doors to check in, to share food, to borrow items, to hang out together. At the same time, there was no lack of drama. The couple two doors down, both of whom I'd befriended, would routinely get into voracious fights and sometimes the police showed up. But they always decided that they loved each other, and things would settle down until the next time. To me, the Manly Building was a microcosm of real life, and I was part of it all.

Several months after moving in, I threw a big party, and it was then and there that I met a woman in a wheelchair, a new resident, who became one of my best friends in life. I could be convinced after a few beers that Laura and I were old souls who'd been connected in the past and now mystically reconnected in the present. Like me, Laura is what uninformed, or maybe "unformed," people would call "handicapped." And I would correct even a whiff of that sentiment by exclaiming, "You've got that wrong—we're "handi-capable!" I think this little play on words is clever and creative; Laura disagrees, calling it jocular but juvenile.

Laura contracted polio as an infant. Although she was able to get around with the aid of special crutches for most of her younger life, she is now confined to a wheelchair. "Confined" is not really a word that fits Laura, however, because she is one of the most high profile, "in your face" athletes in town. You may doubt me until you witness her fly by you at thirty miles per hour on the downhill section of Union Hill.

We very quickly became two peas in a pod, both naturally social, ready to engage in conversation with anyone who crosses our path— a vagrant hipster mooching a cigarette on the sidewalk or the CEO of Peoples United Bank. We are always up for either conversation. We're not afraid to laugh at ourselves and the figure we cut on the sidewalks of Brattleboro. Passersby would never guess I am blind. I look as though I am pushing Laura's wheelchair effortlessly as we traipse along our route, the whole time laughing, singing, snickering, and stopping in at our favorite drop-in spots where we are preferred customers. Because of my blindness and because of Laura's general outlook on the world, we're oblivious to being overheard or any judgments we arouse. Laura trusts no one but me to hoist her, wheelchair and all, up a stairway we need to mount. And I have no greater faith in anyone's opinion about how I look in a pair of shorts I'm considering buying!

*a*SHORTLY AFTER NEIL MOVED INTO the High Street apartment he got word from First Descents that he had been chosen as the recipient of that year's Spirit Award. He was honored and agreed, without hesitation, to fly to Aspen, Colorado, for the annual fundraising gala at a downtown hotel to accept the award and deliver a speech about his experience the previous summer.

First Descents has a unique arrangement regarding camper participation in its programs. Neil had paid not as much as a dime for the week he had spent on the river in Colorado. His room, board, program, and travel expenses had been paid by someone else. In return, the organization asks that those who benefited from that generosity do their best, following their return home, to raise funds in the year ahead to help pay for another young adult living with cancer to attend a camp.

Upon his return, Neil wrote a letter to the members of our large extended family describing his experience and sharing ways in which the organization had touched his life and the lives of other young adults in his position. He explained that although every camper's story is different—their types of cancer and prognoses varied greatly— they all share the same fears, hopes, dreams, and many similar "war stories" of dealing with treatment. Many of Neil's aunts, uncles, cousins, and friends responded generously. In their own ways they had either partici-pated in or followed his journey and had been supportive of us as a family. They were happy to give to an organization that had uplifted Neil.

The annual fundraiser was, of course, a necessary drive to support the organization's mission. Aside from Neil, others would speak that night and give testimonials about the unique niche First Descents has created within the world of cancer management.

Neil was now beyond the point of terror at the thought of speaking in public, but this speech felt big. And Neil had a vision of what he wanted it to be. He was headed to a gala event, an evening of celebration and high spirits. He did not want his speech to reflect the obvious sadness that First Descents had been created to counter balance. He didn't want to deny the hard facts of his own story or those of others, but he wanted his speech to emphasize the diversion and sense of empowerment the organization injects into the lives of those who so need some lightness of being. I sat with him as he expressed that his speech, though still unplanned and unwritten, would be heartfelt but funny and fun.

He set off for Colorado excited to reconnect with Brad, to meet up with "Chunky," one of his favorite fellow campers who lived on the west coast, and to deliver his message to the well heeled guests who would, hopefully, open their hearts and wallets in behalf of this young and vital organization.

Jim and I were home the night of the event. We are two hours ahead of Mountain Time in Colorado, but we were conscious of the clock all evening. At ten o'clock Eastern Time we looked at each other, and I said, "OK—the fund raising gala is about to begin in Aspen. Keep your fingers crossed for Neil!" We were in bed but not yet asleep when the phone rang that evening. I picked it up and immediately set it on speaker.

"Neil!" I said, without even the complementary, "Hello?" "How did it go?"

"Oh my god, Mom!" he gushed. "It was so great! They loved it! It was so hard to wait through dinner. I had to sit there being nervous, not really connected with anybody. The room was so noisy with tons of people buzzing around. It felt confusing. But when I started my speech, I really got into it, and I wasn't nervous. And afterward I felt like a rock star! People just kept raising their paddles to pledge big bucks to First Descents. I'm so proud about how much I helped. I'm so happy!"

"Neil," I gushed, "I feel like I was there! We're so proud of you. I'm so glad you called! Now I know I'll have a good night's sleep, and I hope you do too."

A few days later Jim and I watched the speech on the First Descents website. We felt undeniably nervous as we saw Neil facing a crowd of expectant gala participants. What parent hasn't experienced that fluttery stomach prior to a recital, a tennis match, a school play? You pray your child, no matter how old, will not be let down, disappointed, embarrassed. We watched as Neil addressed the assembled in a down-to-earth, informal manner, weaving humorous anecdotes of his life dealing with both cancer and blindness into his gratitude for and commitment to First Descents. He seemed to be having a ball himself, and the crowd was with him all the way. Cheers erupted as he was finally presented with a hand-made clay trophy of two climbers ascending a steep peak, with a message in braille at its base. The sculpture sits in his studio today where now and then I stop to run my hands over the small human forms climbing to victory.

~

Not long ago I leafed through Neil's files and came across the document of forms that comprised Neil's Individual Professional Development Plan managed by Joe Stein of Vermont Division for the Blind and Visually Impaired and signed by Neil. The plan was started in 2008, soon after Neil left rehab, and ended in 2012 when the goals of the plan had been achieved. Each year new steps were added as others were met. It was in that packet that I saw the plan for The Carroll Center spelled out. My heart filled with gratitude as I leafed through the pages. Before me was the plan for mobility training, for beginning Braille lessons, for training in computer skills, for independent living skills, for support in accessing job skills.

From my now seasoned perspective of being Neil's mother post illness and blindness, of living through more than seven years of adjustment and challenges we never could have envisioned, I could see that we were never as alone as I sometimes, in my lowest moments, had felt. Here before me was a testament of support, both personal and financial, that had caught us in our confusion and despair and had held us with a commitment to forge a new and a good life for Neil. While nothing could ever ease the sorrow and loss and loneliness of waking up to a life of blindness, a life raft had been thoughtfully constructed to ease the transition.

The final step in the plan I scanned that day was to support Neil in his endeavor to become a certified massage therapist, a dream he had been holding for a number of years and a goal which Joe had supported early on by funding his exploration of massage with Chloe Grant.

~

In the winter of 2010, Neil was ready to move forward with finding a massage therapy program that would accept a blind student and be able to adjust curriculum requirements to accommodate his circumstances. Once again, the worry worm embedded itself into my being, intent on settling in unless I routed it out with hard evidence that there was, indeed, such a program and that it offered a space for Neil with generosity and optimism. After a couple of dead ends— a program that sounded interesting but no longer existed and a chilly, less than empathetic reception from a program that we thought could be a good fit— Joe found the right match, and Neil began his studies in the spring of 2010.

The Pyramid Holistic Health Center, located in Rutland, Vermont, was founded by Bill Kelley as a collaborative of more than forty practitioners in the fields of massage therapy, mental health services, and fitness training. The massage certification program designed by Bill was fairly new at the time that Joe Stein was investigating educational opportunities for Neil. It was unique in that it offered the flexibility for all students to progress at the pace that worked for them, given busy lives of work schedules, family responsibilities, distance, and, in Neil's case, disability.

The Center is located in downtown Rutland in a beautiful old three-story brick building. The ground floor houses a new-age store filled with gems, art objects, incense and oils, jewelry, and books, including an impressive array from different spiritual traditions as well as those dedicated to health and wellness. It also houses Pyramid's "crown jewel"— a salt cave which is a heavenly relaxation chamber constructed of thousands of pounds of Himalayan salt which is touted as an anti-inflammatory agent and thought to release negative ions which promote detoxification. The top two floors of the building house conference and practitioners' spaces.

Bill is a visionary, "can-do" kind of guy and, like Brad Ludden, welcomes challenges with optimism and confidence. From the beginning he and the teachers in the massage program were warm and supportive of Neil's goal to enter the profession of massage therapy. All of them were creative thinkers and problem solvers, people who were not intimidated by the uniqueness of Neil's situation. I was the one who transported Neil to and from Pyramid for a year and a half. I got to chat with his instructors between sessions and occasionally filled in on the massage table as a subject for instruction. It was obvious to me that these professionals thought hard about how best to teach Neil. I witnessed them explain and model a technique for him and then change their tack and try a different way. Teaching Neil required them to reflect on effective modes of communication, to be patient with themselves as well as with him, to be flexible and resourceful. They instilled in me faith in the learning process and in my son as an eager, humble, receptive learner. Each of them felt Neil had the makings of an excellent massage therapist, and they voiced their beliefs that Neil's long-held dream had every chance of becoming a reality.

The first weekend of the program was an "intensive"— an introduction to the program and to the Center's holistic philosophy on wellness in general, an overview of the curriculum and the twelve modules of study which would be conducted on-line at the student's own pace, and hands-on workshops on beginning massage techniques. Neil's mobility instructor, Tracy, drove him to Rutland on a Friday and settled him into a motel room where a Center staff member would pick him up and drop him off. I would meet him on Sunday afternoon at the Pyramid building and drive him home.

When I arrived on Sunday, the students were taking turns practicing on subjects who were stretched out on a number of massage tables in a generous sized room on the second floor of the Center. Neil was not practicing when I entered the room. He was seated but had on an apron like all the other students. I called to him. He jumped up, and he called back with his usual unselfconscious, "Mama!" before embracing me in a bear hug. As he introduced me to his new teachers, he seemed upbeat and playful. His mood put me at ease, and I enjoyed the warm welcome I received from everyone, including one of his soon-to-be favorite teachers who waved to me from under a sheet on the nearest table.

On the drive home he shared the events of the weekend. Not surprisingly, there were ups and downs. During a session that featured massage techniques that students watched a teacher demonstrate, Neil had to say, "This is not working for me." At that point, one of the other teachers, another of his soon-to-be favorites, took him aside, got him situated on a table, and, using the tactile sense, demonstrated the lesson for him.

Neil also shared that, not surprisingly, most of the students were rank beginners. He had had the unusual and unique experience of working under the tutelage of Chloe and using his time as a client with Ben as pre-professional learning practices. For more that a year and a half, following his internship with Chloe, he had regularly recruited friends and family members to be his practice subjects. Not only had he gained much experience, he had gained confidence as well.

As soon as Neil began working his way through the twelve study modules of the program, he became hooked. I witnessed the focus and drive that emerged at various points in his life when something caught his interest. Here was the Neil of the tactile braille tiles, the four year old who practiced, over and over, every day, on a rusty little two-wheeler in the day care yard until he had mastered how to ride. His eagerness to learn everything he could about the structure and function of the skeleton and muscle groups of the human body delighted both Jim and me. We sat through many a recitation and synopsis of what he was learning. He did the research he was asked to do, read the material that the others read, sent in the required papers, and received positive feedback, always.

In the end, what the program staff deemed best for instructing Neil in the area of hands-on technique was for him to come separately for instruction with one of them rather than in a group. They were willing to make this special accommodation if we were flexible enough to come at times that fit their personal and professional schedules. Their offer was a generous gift, and we agreed to it immediately. For the next year and a half, Neil and I made monthly journeys to the Center for instruction, and in October of 2011, Neil was presented with a certificate of completion from the program.

*n*THE BIGGEST ASSET OF THE MASSAGE center and its newly formed school was that it enabled students to work independently and move along at a pace that was right for them. During the intensive first weekend we were introduced to the staff, and each one had areas of specialty—Swedish, deep tissue, cupping, and Bill, the director, was the anatomy expert. We were given all the material that we would use throughout the program. Just as promised, everything that was given to the sighted students that weekend was given to me via my computer which I had been told to bring. The only textbook that would not work for me was the Anatomy Coloring Book. To make up for this situation, I was given individual instruction on the subject of anatomy while on the massage table myself or while practicing on a subject under the supervision of my instructors.

I will never forget the experience of being on the table that first weekend of the program as I received a demonstration massage from one of the instructors. Despite my nervousness about embarking on the program, I was utterly blissed out under her hands. I remember thinking that this was something I wanted to spend my life learning and practicing. I suddenly felt that I was in the right place, a feeling that didn't come to me often.

I thoroughly enjoyed working my way through the twelve

consecutive modules of study. One module might take a couple of weeks to complete; some took me a month and some as many as two months. An example of a module I'd delve into would be formally named "Shoulders and Neck." I'd study and respond to in-depth questions regarding this area of anatomy—the name of each muscle, its function, what each is attached to, and the various massage techniques that support the healing and proper alignment of the area. The next module would move me to the study of another area of the body, and I'd find myself immersed in "Feet and Ankles." Modules of study also included general physiology, allergies, ethics, the five different Swedish massage strokes, a technique called "cupping," even the study of marketing and the running of a business.

Regarding the clinical aspect of study, I so appreciated the privilege of being worked with individually. Because of this arrangement I got to work with two of the most amazing therapists in the program. Every massage therapist has his or her own favorite techniques and personal style, a unique relationship to the human body based on scientific knowledge as well as on instinctual beliefs in best practices. Both of these teachers injected me with excitement for the profession and helped me build a foundation of knowledge that has shaped my own practice. Because of their time, their patience, their ingenuity, I, too, have something to offer to those who seek the benefits of body work.

*a*NEIL STAYED IN TOUCH WITH First Descents and

Brad Ludden throughout the year following his kayaking trip and Spirit Award. At some point in their correspondence, Neil shared a dream with Brad that he envisioned for the future: one summer he would join the First Descents staff as a massage therapist and offer his skills to the participants who were dealing with the kinds of profound emotional and physical stress that he, himself, understood.

In his typical expansive thinking, Brad answered, "Why not start now? This coming summer!" Without hesitation, Neil hopped aboard the "make it happen" train. If you are an optimist yourself, a comrade's optimism is contagious, and the energy that bounces back and forth is super-charged. The role the two planned for Neil was a "massage therapy student-in-training staff member" who would offer his skills to participants after a challenging day on the rapids or a day of rock climbing.

On the other end, Neil's massage therapy teachers recognized the unique opportunity that First Descents was affording him. Though the plan constituted "unsupervised" hours of practice, they decided that as long as Neil took adequate input information on clients and had each fill out an evaluation form following a massage, to be reviewed by them upon his return, they could give him their blessing. I was with Neil's two favorite teachers when this conversation occurred, and two emotions welled up in me simultaneously: admiration for their progressive thinking on the matter and confidence as I witnessed their belief that Neil was capable of taking on this special challenge.

Neil was overjoyed. After such a long spell of having

to focus on his own treatment and recovery, of having to start anew on a career plan, his energy, faith, and hard work were paying off. He had a job!

The summer of 2011 was a period of unfolding and expansion for both Neil and me. He had responsibilities to shoulder and places to be. He shipped his portable massage table and his massage chair to Colorado for the first camp. I, who had been a Nervous Nellie regarding Neil traveling alone, who had always tried to book non-stop flights the few times Neil had flown since his blindness, had to let go and have faith that it would all work out. Throughout that summer, as he traveled back and forth from Vermont to Colorado, Montana, and Oregon, First Descents booked his flights, and all of them had layovers. And, low and behold, he managed. The airlines, I learned, take excellent care of their disabled passengers.

Sometimes Neil would meet and connect with passengers along the way, sometimes not. But every time Jim and I met a plane in order to drive him home, he would come ambling down the corridor on the arm of an airport employee, always the last one off the plane, and they would be chatting, joking, laughing. And every time, whether his guide was an elderly man or a young woman, he or she would greet me, "So, you're Neil's mom!" and inevitably offer a statement along these lines—"This is some guy!" And what could I say but, "I know!"

*n*FOR ME, GETTING THE GIG AT First Descents was tantamount to winning the lottery! I had had the time of my life during my first experience as a participant on the white water kayaking trip on the Colorado River. While I was on this epic adventure, I bonded with Brad and was really moved by the other incredible adult campers. We were all dealing with cancer, but we were all out kayaking or rock climbing together, confirming that life was not over. I remember feeling so high when I came back from that trip. I knew exactly what I wanted to do. I wanted to be a massage therapist working at the First Descents summer programs. I wanted to combine my two passions—practicing massage and getting outdoors to do bad-ass outdoor activities. This would be my dream come true if it ever came to pass. It seemed like a pipe dream, but when I finally got the courage to present the idea to Brad, he was totally on board, as if he'd already been thinking about it himself. I was just finishing my massage therapy course work, so the timing was perfect. Here before me was the most amazing stepping stone to the professional life I was working toward!

My teachers took a risk on me. They realized that the clients I would encounter constituted a specialty population: they were living with cancer somewhere within their bodies. But my teachers also acknowledged that each participant was hale enough, at this point, to engage in challenging physical endeavors, and they realized that I, myself, was a member of that group. I shared a similar life. I was a massage therapist-in-training-with empathy. I might not know clients' individual cancer scenarios, but I knew their stress, their grief, and their fear.

That summer, the camper/clients who came to me for massage

knew about my own cancer story, and they expressed their admiration that I was in the midst of writing my personal "Chapter Two" after "Chapter One" of my life was behind me for good.

They were very open to having body work. I let them know that I could offer some relief and that they, in turn, were giving me the practice I needed to move forward in my new profession and my new life. Throughout the summer I worked on young people who have since passed away and on those whose cancers were not life-threatening and are now completely healthy. I offered massage during a three hour period each evening. During the day I could go out and participate in the same activities they were doing and experience the same adventures. When they came in for massage, I could say, "You were unbelievable out in the rapids today," or "You really aced it on the rock this afternoon," because many days I was among them. And now I got to be the therapy guy and offer a different, additional mode of healing. For me, it couldn't get much better than that. The whole package was my privilege, my pleasure.

FOURTEEN

SHELTER

"There's no place like home!"

~ Dorothy, *The Wizard of Oz*

*a*NEIL LIVED IN THE MANLY BUILDING on High Street for almost two years before it became evident that his needs had changed, and it was time to move on. Both he and I still loved the straightforward, spacious physical space as much as ever, but little things began to bug me. And different issues nagged at him.

For me, the issue of having to pay for parking every time I dropped by was wearing thin. The parking fees in the public lot abutting his building were the cheapest in town, but it was still a pain to sift through my change every time I wanted to drop something off or to make sure I'd paid enough if I wanted to stay for a more extended visit. In addition, it had become annoying hauling heavy grocery bags across the lot, up the steps, and down a long hallway before we got to his kitchen. I couldn't see us doing this forever.

But the biggest drawback was this: there was absolutely

no outdoor space. If Neil had had a small yard to enjoy when the weather was warm and pleasant or a porch to sit on and feel the breeze or the sunshine, it would have made a big difference in the quality of his life. When he was at home, however, he was pretty much trapped indoors.

Neil had wanted an apartment in the downtown area, but the truth is that he rarely walked the sidewalks alone. Crossing streets, even ones with auditory aids, remained challenging, and his accuracy in keeping a straight line across the crosswalk was unpredictable. Going out with a companion was just more relaxing, more fun.

Neil did not complain of the "trapped inside" issue. He may not have felt it as much as I did, vicariously, or he might not have wanted to call attention to his limitations in the area of mobility. But, in my mind, having a yard with safe access or a connected porch or deck would afford him a freedom he currently lacked—the ability to be outdoors whenever he wanted without help from others. And for me, Neil's freedom and independence were always the goals.

When Neil first moved into his apartment, part of the pleasure of being in the building was that he met several neighbors his age with whom he visited back and forth. They became part of the fabric of his social life. They had easy access to each other. Over time, however, one by one, for various reasons, these fellow apartment dwellers moved out and on to new phases of their lives. And no one who subsequently moved into their vacated apartments ever took their places in Neil's day to day life. It's just the way it played out. But, to me, a message seemed to be emerging: "pay tribute to and feel gratitude for a stage of life that engendered growth but recognize that it may have been a stepping stone to the next chapter."

In the end, what propelled Neil to move on from the Manly Building was his drive to start his own business following his successful completion of his certification program. He needed a site in a highly visible location with easy access for clients. And he needed to be on site, himself, so that being present for appointments never depended on transportation issues. What he needed was a house.

～

The clarity that Neil needed a massage studio within his own home came after a disappointing plan-in-the-making with another massage therapist. She owned a small store-front studio and natural health and beauty products shop on the parking lot side of Neil's building. They had been introduced to each other and connected over the fact that Neil had just completed his certification program and was looking for a suitable venue to embark on his new profession. She asked Neil to give her a massage, then demonstrate an additional massage on her co-worker. Following the two massages she expressed her enthusiasm about his skill. After several chats over coffee, she asked him to join her practice as she was busy with other aspects of the business and needed more time at home with her child.

Both Neil and Jim were ecstatic. In contrast, I didn't understand the plan. The arrangement seemed way too vague.

"What does this entail?" I asked. "How do you and she decide which clients to take? How do you become known? Are you supposed to be in the shop when she's not there? What do you do when you are there without a client? You said the space was very tight. Does that work for you? Are you supposed to stay home until you are called to give a massage, then go down for an hour?"

I had an unsettled feeling about it. Neil was concerned that the percentage of money she proposed to take from his work was too high. In the end, none of these specific questions mattered. The massage therapist contacted him and, without explanation, told him that she had changed her mind about her offer. She felt that this merger was not a good match for her.

Neil was devastated. Such disappointments are difficult for any of us. They submerge us in the murky waters of doubt about our abilities, our confidence in who we are, and what we have to offer. It's hard to be in that place ourselves and just as hard to shepherd a loved one through it.

"Neil," I tried explaining to him. "This kind of thing happens to all of us in life. And it's hard not to, but we just can't take it so personally. And there is such a thing as 'not the right match.'"

But I felt his pain. Feeling rejected is no fun, and being reminded that it is a universal human experience doesn't help much when the hurt is newly inflicted. It takes time to gain some perspective and wisdom about it all.

But, in the end, this event was the catalyst for Neil to embark on his own: to create a business with a web site and business cards and local advertising and his own sign hanging from his own porch, welcoming the public to his place of business within his new home.

THE MANLY BUILDING WAS MY home for two years—two important years. It was there that I practiced and put to use the skills of independence I had learned at The Carroll Center. And it was there that I met for the first time people who had not known me before becoming blind. The Neil they met and spent time with was the only Neil they'd ever known. But, after a while, the fit was not quite right. I likened it to trying on a new pair of slightly tight shoes. You convince yourself that they are really OK—comfortable, even. But eventually, as time goes on, those few tight spots become more noticeable, less forgiving, until you experience undeniable friction that leads to blisters.

As much as I loved my apartment as a general living space, my goal was to practice massage therapy. During the year and a half that I'd studied to earn my certificate, I had offered friends and acquaintances free massages to accrue as much practice as possible between my sessions at the Pyramid School. I had set up my massage table in my living room, pulled the blinds for privacy, and turned on peaceful music. But it was obvious that my apartment was not suitable for a studio. It would have been awkward for potential repeat clients to return regularly to my living room for hour long, paid massages.

As a solution to my dilemma, I contacted a massage therapist who was located on the first floor side entrance to my building. She operated a storefront featuring skin care products, and included within the store was a small massage space. She not only was receptive but seemed excited about the possibility of my joining her practice. She asked me to give her a sample massage and also to demonstrate my technique on her employee. As she oriented me through the store to the table, I wondered how I was ever going to move deftly around the space. But, outwardly, I displayed nothing but excitement at the prospect of starting my first job in my new profession and working with her.

Both the owner and the employee seemed to enjoy their massages, with sighs of relaxation and murmurs of release as I located and worked on the tight spots that plague us all. Following this initial test, I was asked to bring in two more people so the owner could continue to observe and assess my practice. I chose my brother-in-law Kurt who was visiting for Christmas and a female friend whose apartment was two doors down from mine. Everything went well as I skirted my way carefully around the table. I left feeling great about my performance and let go of my reservations about the small work space. I was sure I'd adjust and learn to feel at home in it.

The evening before I was due to formally start the job I got a call from my new massage therapy colleague. She said that she had reconsidered her offer and had changed her mind.

I should look elsewhere for a position. I couldn't believe it! I had jumped through so many hoops! Had I completely misread the feedback she'd given me? How could I have been so off target? When I asked about what had changed her mind, where I had fallen down, she responded that she'd decided that the fit just wasn't right. And that was that.

I had a hard time coming to terms with the fact that I'd been fired before I was formally hired! I felt a tremendous letdown on the heels of such a sudden and confusing rejection and was plagued by not knowing what I had done wrong. Was it my skill level? Did I not, literally, fit into the tiny studio? Did the owner decide that my blindness was too difficult a situation to deal with?

Ironically, this blow turned out to be the impetus to make a huge change in my life. My focus was to become a successful massage therapist. I had been rejected, possibly due to my disability, and my current apartment was holding me back. The apartment had already overpaid its dues. I couldn't have lived in a better location or building during my orientation to a whole new way of being in the world. But now I'd outgrown it. While it was hard to imagine leaving my home behind, it was time to look at what the future had in store.

TOGETHER, NEIL, JIM, AND I BEGAN brainstorming ideas for next steps in our connected lives. What did Neil want? What did we, as Neil's parents and primary emotional supporters, want for him? What did Jim and I want for ourselves? The answers to these questions needed to be clarified as we moved forward.

Neil was clear that he wanted to be a massage therapist. It was his calling, and he had never wavered from his desire to pursue this dream nor his decision that this was the right path for him. In addition, his goal was to once again be part of the work force. While he knew he would probably always need help in the form of his disability income, he was eager to contribute to his livelihood to the best of his ability. And, last, but essential to acknowledge: work gives most of us a sense of identity, an anchor that helps us describe to ourselves and others a part of who we are.

Like most good parents, Jim's and my most fervent hope is that our children have happy and fulfilling lives. None of us has control over the turn of events and the way life unfolds. If we ever, subconsciously, believed in a modicum of cosmic influence, that veil had been lifted the day we learned that Neil had been living with a tumor secretly smoldering deep inside his brain. What we could do, however, was to live large, take appropriate risks, and give whatever we had to give. And Jim and I as a team have never doubted this way of being in the world. Gradually, a vision, a picture, began to emerge before us. We would try to find a house, buy it, and rent it to Neil.

≈

Our first glimpse of the house that was to be Neil's was online.

Jim called me from his perch in front of the laptop where he had been scouting properties for rent or sale in Brattleboro.

"Honey, come and look at this place. It's a foreclosure, bank owned, and the price is right."

I peered over his shoulder at what looked like a little, red New England farmhouse with a white-railed front porch. It sat close to the sidewalk on High Street, the same street on which Neil's apartment building was located, still within walking distance of downtown but set among a cluster of residences, some which were occupied by families, some which housed the offices of law, dental, and real estate businesses. I knew this area to be "curb-appeal" lovely. It was a great location for both living, if you didn't mind being on a busy, main street, and running a business, which could only benefit from being on a busy main street! The house was advertised as a multi-unit but one that could easily be converted back to single-unit.

"Wow," I ventured, "I love it from the outside, but it must be in really rough shape inside, or it wouldn't be selling at that price. It obviously didn't start out as a multi-unit home. I'll bet it's chopped up in a weird way inside. Probably, over the years, there's been a heavy turnover of occupants."

"Let's drive by," shot Jim, ignoring my musings on the probable shortcomings of the property. "We have errands to do in Brattleboro anyway."

My radar is activated when Jim is on a quest. I know the signs. He becomes highly enthusiastic and sprouts blinders to possible roadblocks. He is always sure he can find ways around them, ways that are not obvious to other, more measured thinkers.

I recognize that this quality in him has been an attraction to me all along our journey together. However, I often play the devil's advocate. It's an important role to play in any major decision. Sometimes I am right, and together we pull back. But many times over the years I have been swept away by Jim's enthusiasm. It's like gaining cosmic permission to think bigger than I ordinarily would. I step outside the small me into the bigger me who is always there but not always confident to shine forth. And when I'm on board, I become a major player. My energies, both creative and physical, soar. I am lit from within.

But nothing could have prepared me for the interior of 160 High Street that afternoon in late December. We pulled up in front of the house that we had driven by hundreds of times in our travels to and from Brattleboro. With eyes on the road ahead, a driver couldn't possibly take in all the residences that flanked this lovely tree-lined street which emptied onto Main Street with its shops, restaurants, and art galleries. The house was not flashy. It sat quietly, diminutively, between a well-kept taller home and a grand but faded Mary Poppins-style house turned apartment building. The house looked just as sweet as it had in the online photo— a little down at the mouth but classic in its lines and proportions. We climbed out of the car. Jim walked the sidewalk back and forth several times, examining its street-side exterior from every angle. I scrambled onto the porch to peek in a window. Before I could cup my hands and press them like binoculars against the glass, however, I heard voices from within.

"Oh, no," I hissed to Jim, keeping my voice as low as

possible, "there are people inside. Maybe they're striking a deal right now, and this place will be off the market by tomorrow!"

Jim, by nature more reserved than I am in situations in which he feels we may be overstepping our bounds, implored me to get off the porch and into the car. I hesitated, then gave in to his request. I turned around in retreat and told myself I'd call the listing agency the following day. But before I reached the car, the front door opened. I swung around and came face to face with an attractive woman about my age with a head of stunning white hair tied back into a pony tail.

"Oh hi," I mumbled sheepishly. "Are you looking at the house?"

"No," she answered, "I'm showing it."

I don't know what emboldened me or what made me blurt out an unrehearsed, thought-free request. It just flew out of my mouth.

"Can we come in too?"

She didn't hesitate, just pulled the door open wider, stepped to the side, and answered, "Yes."

I called down to Jim on the sidewalk, "The realtor said we could come in!"

As he shook his head, no, I turned my back on him and walked through the door. There are times I follow Jim, and, just as often, there are times he has no choice but to follow my headstrong lead.

We entered a hallway covered in an old-fashioned wallpaper, now faded and nondescript. To the left I caught a glimpse of the living room, but straight ahead the hallway dead-ended in a wall covered in the same tired paper. Though the proportions of the hall were pleasing, the fact that it lead to nowhere made it less attractive than it would have been had there been the view of a welcoming room beyond it. It puzzled me until a realization dawned. It HAD once lead into a room, a room that must have had two points of entry. The only reason I could imagine walling off this entry would be to construct a hall closet. But that had not been done. Nowhere in the hall was a space to hang a coat or leave winter boots. To the right, a sturdy staircase covered in a handsome Oriental carpet rose to the second floor. I felt encouraged.

We turned left and walked into the living room. It was a dingy shade of salmon. The ceiling displayed several deep cracks, and there were a few gauges in the walls, but the room had a spacious square shape. The white trim on the four windows had a solid but graceful look. The sides were beveled, and the tops rose to a peak. The room pleased me. I could see its charm, and I knew that it wouldn't take much to make it beautiful again.

I glimpsed the kitchen from the back wall of the living room. I admired how the transition from living room to kitchen did not feel chopped up like in other homes of this vintage where the passage between rooms is a standard, narrow doorway. This passage was triple wide, more like a generous arch. There was a nearly full view of the kitchen from the living room. I grinned. It was an old fashioned version of today's "open plan!"

I headed eagerly for the archway to take in the kitchen,

and it was there and then that my heart sank. I felt as if I were standing on a bridge: behind me lay potential and before me, despair.

The room was rife with grunge factor. I could barely acknowledge its good points: its spacious, square proportions; its huge tract of U-shaped Formica counter; its row of obviously hand-made cabinets. Several of the greasy dark cabinet doors listed drunkenly on a single hinge just waiting for those tired hinges to lose hold and slam them to the floor. Brittle, food-stained contact paper clung tenaciously to every interior cabinet shelf. The once white-patterned linoleum floor was mottled gray and brown, its four edges curling inward in a seeming race to beat each other to the center of the room. There was no refrigerator or stove, but two dirty, empty spaces revealed their former positions. Short of a complete gutting and an entire renovation, which I knew was financially impossible for us, I was not sure where I would start. As I stood there, that heady creative swirling which had enveloped me moments before as I assessed the hallway and living room evaporated.

And things got worse. This house was much larger than we had imagined. Like many New England farm-style houses, this seemingly small house stretched way out the back. There were two more rooms beyond the kitchen and another directly off the kitchen, the one that had been blocked from the front hallway—the only room that bumped out from the long straight footprint of the house.

The two rooms at the back were smaller that the front

rooms, and both had doorways leading onto a spacious deck overlooking the small, overgrown yard I had dreamed about. It was obvious that these back rooms and two small upstairs rooms, reached by a small winding stairway, had been part of a now defunct apartment. The furthest room was the roughest. One of its mustard colored walls was streaked with grease, and several naked pipes emerged from underneath the floor boards. There was no sink nor any appliances, but it was evident that this room must have been the apartment's kitchen. The drop ceiling overhead was buckling.

Off the room was a bathroom that would have elicited squeamishness in anyone. Floor tiles were chipped and mismatched; the cheap tub surround was streaked with soap scum; and the toilet was sinking into the floorboards below the tile. The wood was obviously rotting due to a hidden leak. Nevertheless, this final room had its charm. I loved the horizontal bead board walls. Its position far from the street gave it the feel of quiet seclusion, and the windows let in ample light.

As we worked our way back to the kitchen, we turned left through a doorway and entered the large "bump-out" room. I noticed immediately that two of its three windows practically hugged the side of the neighboring house, shockingly close for comfort. Its claustrophobic feeling was heightened by the fact that the walls were painted dark blue. The floor was covered in a wall to wall shag that I later dubbed "Grover" blue after the Sesame Street puppet. At one end of the room was a small lavatory which contained a tiny old fashioned sink, a window that blessed the space with natural light, and a high end toilet that sat a little crookedly as one side was sinking through the floor. Despite its problems, the little lavatory held its own: I loved it straight away.

We circled the room separately, Jim attempting to poke through a sagging ceiling tile to determine what disaster it was meant to camouflage, me toying with window treatment ideas that would keep the neighbors from voyeurism, even if that was the last thing on their minds. We met back in the center of the room, and suddenly I felt a wave of inspiration. The room had revealed itself to me without my consciously knowing it.

"Jim," I said softly, but I could feel my enthusiasm expand and grow stronger as I gave voice to the message for which I was the channel. "This is the perfect massage studio! It has its own little bathroom; the windows facing the neighbor's house could be sheathed in white curtains that let in light but no view. People who come for massages want complete privacy and a feeling of safe enclosure, and that's exactly what this room provides. We could close off the doorway from the kitchen and re-open the wall that leads to the front hall. That way clients could come in the front door and enter the massage room without ever going through Neil's living space. Can you picture it? Tell me what you think!"

We walked around again with the vision percolating. Jim probed the solid wall which blocked off the hallway, giving silent thought to my idea. I understood that he couldn't give the wall more that a quick, cursory once-over and wouldn't be able to proclaim my plan a "sure thing." But I felt heartened when he announced that he didn't think the wall was an essential bearing wall, impossible to remove.

We worked our way back through the kitchen, the living room, the hall, and up the staircase to the second floor. At the top of the stairs, to the right, was a huge full bathroom. The floor was sheathed in two different pieces of linoleum; one lay on top of the other, most likely to create a patch where needed. The tub was heavy and generous but badly stained. The handmade vanity was constructed of cheap plywood and awkwardly placed within the room.

"Wow," said Jim in a low voice. "I'd have to measure this space to be sure, but if we bought a new vanity and moved it over to the left, I think the perpendicular wall would be long enough to hold both a washer and dryer."

I stood close to him in order to hear his low decibel musings. I knew why he was speaking in a near whisper. From one of the bedrooms we could hear the two somewhat unsavory-looking guys who had actually made an appointment to view the house. The realtor had been generous with them as well as with us. She wasn't actually "showing" any of us the house. She was letting us wander about and discover it for ourselves. What, after all, were the highlights she wanted us to focus on? What attributes were obvious selling points? She was simply present to answer questions. She knew exactly what to do and how to be, and I appreciated her. I listened as these two were trying to figure how to further cut up the house, how to change it from a two-unit to a three-unit dwelling in order to gain an additional rent. "Poor House," I thought to myself. "If you thought you were going to be rescued and loved, I don't think that's in the cards if these dudes have their way."

As the men made their way back downstairs to review the sequence of rooms and conjure possible configurations to support their plan, Jim and I entered the bedroom opposite the bathroom. It had wow factor in that it was huge with two windows overlooking High Street.

"This is where a bed should go," I pointed to Jim.

"Uh-huh," he agreed, "And Neil could have his Elliptical Runner between the two windows It's unbelievable to find a bedroom big enough for a workout machine. It's a perfect space. The Elliptical wouldn't be in the way of anything."

But the room, as well as a smaller bedroom across the hall, also had plenty of ugh factor. Both had faded, stained wallpaper, and both were wall-to walled with the same Grover-blue shag that covered the bump-out room downstairs. Every square inch of the rooms screamed, "Work!"

The two small back rooms which had been the upstairs of the former apartment felt very separate from the main upstairs. They were not in bad shape, needed some spit and polish, and lacked adequate electrical outlets. We certainly didn't need them, and making use of them was beyond the scope of our thinking at that point.

All in all, the house had nine rooms—more than we bargained for—and most in need of major overhaul. As we pulled away from High Street and headed north to Westminster West, I attempted to recreate in my mind what I'd just seen. I tried to walk the blueprint. But I couldn't. It was a chaotic morass that swirled haphazardly in my memory. I couldn't remember which room led into which room. I didn't recall whether the small, winding back staircase was in the furthest downstairs back room or the middle back room. I tried to group the dizzying swirl of images into two categories—positive and negative. I opened to the house's potentials: its overall size, its individual spaces, its deck and yard, its undeniably perfect location. But I couldn't hold on. My mind shifted to images of sagging ceilings and floors, of every surface being broken, stained, faded, cracked, grimy, old, and undeniably ugly. The scale tipped steeply, and I slid into the negative.

For the first couple of miles neither Jim nor I spoke. We sat with our own private thoughts. But, finally, I shared what was on my mind.

"I guess you get what you pay for. We're certainly not going to buy that place!"

I waited for Jim to take his turn. He looked straight ahead at the road and answered, "Actually, yes, we are."

❧

The day following our unplanned viewing of the house we took Neil to see it in his own way. Once again, the low-key realtor respectfully occupied herself as Jim walked about taking videos of each space, accompanied by audio observations, and Neil and I threaded our way through the hallway, living room, kitchen, and the room I'd envisioned as the massage studio. He seemed as enthusiastic about his spatial and tactile impressions of the house as he had been when we described it to him the night before. Enthusiasm is "catching" after all. I had ended up catching it from Jim, and I hoped Neil would catch it from me.

He and I climbed the staircase to the second floor, turned right to explore the bathroom, then entered the bedroom that would be his. After his initial perusal of the room, I brought him back to the space between the two street-side windows.

"Neil, Dad and I thought this would be the ideal place for your Elliptical. And right across from it," (I pulled him to the opposite wall), "right here, would be the perfect placement for your bed. Can you picture it?"

"I think I can," he said, "but this has totally been enough for right now. I don't want to know anything about the guest room or the upstairs and downstairs back rooms. This is plenty for me to work with and memorize."

And he was right. The spaces we covered were completely adequate for his personal and professional needs. There was no need for more. Squeezing his hand, I agreed with him. He squeezed back. I knew he was excited, but I sensed that he was equally overwhelmed from the effort of taking on the unfamiliar without benefit of sight.

"Neil," I said, "I'm so glad you like the house, and I know you're going to love living here. I just get the feeling that this is a happy house."

"So do I, Mom," he answered with his signature winning smile, "and before we leave, let's do the tour one more time!"

~

We explained to Neil that although the house at 160 High Street had potential and possibilities—he might, down the line, want to rent one of the back rooms to another complementary body work professional—it was currently in a sorry state and needed both structural and cosmetic work. It was in no way move-in ready. Right now it was a project of grand proportions.

Neil's response was optimistic. "We can do it! We'll have fun, and I want to be part of everything as much as I can. I know there are some jobs I can do. I want to help restore the house that's going to be mine."

Jim and I closed on the house at 160 High Street in late January, 2012, just days before we were set to drive to Florida for the month of February. The timing wasn't great. Our travel plans meant postponing the start of the monumental project which would render the house habitable for Neil and for his business. But our plans were non-negotiable. Before we left, we made plans with a plumber and an electrician to begin work the week we arrived home. We left a key to the house with Neil. Every few days that February he made plans to show the house to a friend or relative. And each trip gave him further practice in memorizing the footprint of his new digs.

Almost everyone agrees that moving is an arduous, no-fun task. And I have this to add: moving is doubly hard when you are blind. While I knew I had outgrown my apartment in the Manly Building—it no longer met my needs in too many ways—it felt like a major leap to abandon all that I had become accustomed to. When you are blind, especially newly blind, your own house is the only place you feel completely comfortable and in control. Issues that sighted people do not need to overly focus on—whether their bedside table is truly a mere hand's reach away; deciding which plate or utensil goes to the right or left in which cupboard or drawer; choosing and sticking to the same spot on the bathroom counter to park your toothbrush and toothpaste; remembering which area of which shelf holds pants as opposed to shirts—these seemingly minor details are hugely important in the world of a blind person. Eyesight is the God-given tool for mapping the environment, figuring out the lay of the land, locating a needed item with just a glance. Groping hands are a sorry substitution.

Since becoming blind, I have learned the hard lesson that organization is key to making life run as smoothly as possible. It was not easy for me to make this adjustment. In my former life, everything went wherever I happened to leave it, and just because I became blind overnight didn't mean that I did or could immediately become an organized person. But, ultimately, I had no choice. I slowly and consciously, starting in my parents' home and then in my own apartment, made the transition from my old habits to a life of purposeful organization. After all the work of this transition and of eventually feeling like a competent master of my now-familiar environment, it was not surprising that fear rose up in me at the thought of leaving it all and starting again in a new space. Although my apartment had its restrictions in terms of my future plans, I had committed it to memory, knew it without having to stop and think. I realized that staying there would hold me back from my goal of opening my own massage therapy studio, but mixed feelings are part of trading one good thing for another.

∾

I had no part in finding my new residence. My mother and I had had a number of conversations about the advantages of moving on, but the actual doing of it lay somewhere "out there," comfortably removed from NOW. As I was processing the idea, getting my head around the prospect that this might actually happen, my folks stumbled upon a house that interested them. It was a foreclosure, a ramshackle house that had been uninhabited for four years. It was located on High Street, the same street as my apartment building but in a neighborhood setting. Its location was "primo" as both a residence for me and as a highly visual, accessible site to run a small business.

When my parents took me on the initial tour, I could feel the aura of neglect and abandonment emanating from the rooms. They had a sort of medieval dungeon feel. Most of the rooms had wall-to-wall carpets that smelled as though the former occupant was one of those old ladies who harbored three dozen cats and didn't believe in litter boxes. My mother described the walls' dark colors, and her visual cues further heightened my image of a less than welcoming interior. The electricity had been disconnected years ago, and the kitchen sink didn't release a drop of water. As I tracked my hand along the wall of one of the back rooms, I felt what I recognized as a random array of stickers of various shapes and sizes. They now seemed permanently cemented to the wall where a little kid probably slept or played. I cringed when I thought of the poor schmuck who soon would have to scrape them off. Then I realized that that might, in fact, be me. In all honesty, my mind wavered back and forth between enthusiasm and doubt during my first tour, but, in the end, enthusiasm won out. I had all the faith in the world in my father's judgment and his vision, so I climbed gamely on board and applauded my parents' willingness to make an offer that no man, or in this case, no bank could refuse.

In short order we became the proud owners of 160 High Street. Immediately following the closing my parents took off for a well-deserved winter retreat in Florida. The day before they departed on their long drive down the east coast, my father handed me the key to my future home. I worked the common little key around in my hand, rubbing my thumb over its hole and feeling its pattern of jagged edges with my index finger. Suddenly I felt as though this was not just any key. I was holding the key to my new life. As I hugged my parents good-bye, I told them how excited I was and how I hoped they weren't sick of hearing me repeat, for the umpteenth time, how much gratitude and love I had for them both. They laughed, and Dad said, "Let's just agree that you owe us eternally!" Mom encouraged me to take my friends on grand tours around the place, not only to show it off but to familiarize myself with it again and again so that I would memorize it as I'd done with my apartment.

And that is exactly what I did. Any friends or acquaintances I could talk into checking out my new place endured one of the worst Open House tours ever. Some saw the potential and marveled that nine rooms were hiding behind its deceptively small street-side exterior. Others did their best to feign excitement for me as they tried not to make contact with the grimy walls. A couple of my closest friends endured the tour more than once, for my sake, and patiently helped reorient me when I got turned around and hopelessly confused.

UPON OUR RETURN, JIM AND I worked on the interior of 160 High Street seven days a week until Neil officially moved in on the first of May 2012. We lived and breathed the project all of March and April, working on our individual, designated jobs in parallel play with each other and taking turns partnering with Neil on some major tasks. We made decisions as we went along, then shopped for the building supplies, hardware, paint, and lighting fixtures to implement those decisions. We were swept up in a zone of creative energy, of problem-solving, of collaboration, of negotiating with each other about what we could afford to spend money on and what we could not.

Jim's role, given his background, was far more complicated and diverse than mine. His experience, both as a carpenter and a general contractor was, without question, the only reason we could attempt taking this sow's ear of a house and labor to transform it into a warm, welcoming home and place of business. While we shared the vision equally, it was his knowledge and experience that were the foundation of the project. My specialty was that of a persistent, hard-working, unskilled laborer. And there were no lack of projects of that variety at 160 High Street in the spring of 2012. Scrubbing, scraping, sanding, painting—those were the jobs with my name on them.

"OK, Neil," I proclaimed a day after we arrived home from Florida. "You and I are going to start on the kitchen. "Dad is going to unscrew all these old cabinet doors and deposit them in the back room. I'm going to start peeling and scraping all the contact paper from the cabinet shelves, both above the counters and below. And you are going to scrub down all the cabinet frames, uppers and lowers. Here's a bucket of hot water and Murphy's Oil Soap. If we don't wash off every streak of grease or grime, I'm afraid the paint won't stick. Are you down for this job?"

"Absolutely," he answered without hesitation. "And, Mom, how about listening to a little reggae as we work?"

And so we began. It was a perfect job for Neil. Feeling the exterior frames of the cupboards with the doors removed and moving down the line with his sponge was a straightforward task. It was the kind of linear, tactile job that proved successful for him. It was an essential first step in reclaiming and reusing what we'd inherited in the kitchen, and Neil was the right man for the job.

Following our scraping and cleaning, we both painted. I hunched and reached with my brush into the interior of each cupboard, and Neil started down the line of frames again, trading a sponge for a brush.

"Neil!" I proclaimed, standing back to assess our work. "This creamy white paint has improved the kitchen already. It's so bright and clean looking!"

"I know, Mom," he answered, "I can see it."

The next step in our project was tackling the cupboard doors, uppers and lowers. There were twenty-four in all! I set Neil up on a lawn chair in the room outside the kitchen. Directly in front of him was a make-shift table—two saw horses bridged by a piece of plywood.

"OK, Buddy," I began, "here's a piece of sandpaper, and by your left foot is a stack of cupboard doors. Just do a quick sanding on the front and back of each and move the one you've finished over to your right. I've got my own sandpaper and stack as well. We're doing the same job, and with the two of us working it shouldn't take long."

We sat, we chatted, we listened to music, and sang along. And just as sweet, we were making progress.

The winter of 2012 was an unusual one in New England: it was a rare La Niña year of uncharacteristically warm days. The high temps did not last throughout the spring, but the first two weeks of March were downright balmy, a boon for two sanders, now turned painters, confronting the backs and fronts of twenty-four cupboard doors. I moved our identical saw-horse stations outside to the deck where each of us could suspend a door, back-side first, coat it with stain-sealing primer, then flip it onto its front and do the same. We couldn't believe we were outdoors in our shirtsleeves in March! When Neil finished painting a side, he'd announce, "Done, Mom," and I would glance at it and either say, "Good job, flip it over," or reach over with my brush, swipe an area he'd missed and tell him, "OK, you're ready to flip." We proceeded this way over days and days, some of them indoors when the weather turned cold. We painted the front of each cupboard door three times, once with primer and twice with a serene blue-gray paint, and the back of each with one coat of primer and one top coat.

"Neil," I announced one day toward the end of this marathon, "each cupboard door has received five coats of paint, and we've painted twenty-four of them. That's one hundred twenty coats in all."

"No wonder I'm sick of it," he answered.

"You and me, both," I shot back.

~

At last the cupboard doors were hung on their original hinges. Although we had planned to replace the old brass hinges—they were dull and spotted with age—their very narrow size was impossible to duplicate. None of the hardware stores and outlets had hinges the width we needed. Jim ended up having to fish them out of the trash bin and took on the task of cleaning and polishing all forty-eight of them. It was labor intensive, but as he sat in the living room lawn chair scrubbing away, I cheered him on. We were reusing and recycling. The house would have a new life with nods to its past, and it was a thought that appealed to both of us.

In mid-April I took a break and flew to North Carolina. Jessica had just given birth to our grandson, Luke, and I couldn't wait to be by their side. Jim stayed behind with Neil to continue moving forward on the house. I returned five days later, in love with our new grandson and happy with the knowledge that Jessica, her husband Kurt, and baby Luke would take up residence in Vermont for most of the coming summer. Kurt, an experienced carpenter, was willing to arrange his schedule in order to begin work on the exterior of Neil's house. Jim would meet his new grandson in six weeks time.

Jim and I picked Neil up for work on the morning following my return.

"We have a surprise for you," Jim announced as we pulled into the driveway. "Let's go in the front door this morning."

We stepped onto the sagging front porch where I'd stood, in peeking mode, just a couple of months earlier, and Neil said, "OK, Mom, shut your eyes."

Together they led me into the front hall. We stopped, and on command I opened my eyes to take in their surprise. Before me was a new door, a beautiful, paneled, golden oak door that led from the hallway into Neil's massage studio—the door I had envisioned on my first visit to this shabby, forlorn house.

"I love it!" I said over and over again. "Tell me everything, the whole door saga that took place while I was gone!"

"Well," started Jim, "I knew it was a two-man job, everything from loading the behemoth onto our truck and carrying it inside to Neil holding it level while I worked on the installation. Neil's the one who nailed down all the trim. We think it came out pretty well, and we couldn't wait to show you!"

"It's better than I envisioned," I exclaimed. "This is a more beautiful door than I imagined. It's the first thing you see when you open the front door. It gives the hallway a sense of purpose that it so needed."

"Good!" replied Neil.

I could tell that Jim, too, was pleased by my reaction, but with his trademark modesty, he laughed and proclaimed, "And, onto the next..."

～

The project of renovating Neil's new home was a bonding experience for the three of us. And if we'd had time to be introspective, which we couldn't really afford during those whirlwind days, we might have seen that the experience provided us a close-up of each other's basic natures—the shape and texture of our individual fortitude, resilience, approaches, senses of humor. And if, for some reason, those days represented a kind of cosmic test,

I'd have to say that we all passed with flying colors because, true to Neil's prediction, we had a really, really, really good time.

*n*IN A MONTH'S TIME MY PARENTS returned home, and we went to work with the assistance of a plumber, an electrician, and the window installer who replaced every one of the lead-painted windows within two days' time. My dad, of course, was chief carpenter, and I was his willing assistant. I was anxious to do everything I could to help in the effort, and both he and my mother included me in jobs that lent themselves to my altered skill level. My brother-in-law Kurt, an experienced carpenter, came up from North Carolina that summer to work on the exterior of the house. Rounding out the team was the most talented and hardest working interior designer in the business: my mother. With my sister and me as her assistants, we repainted every room in the house. After Mom and Jessica decided on a lighter, more cheerful and uplifting color, we would go to work. They took on the walls and trim of each room, and I would be assigned to paint the inner walls of its accompanying closet. They assured me that closets were of the utmost importance—they would only be painted once in a lifetime and would be highly scrutinized, so I joyfully complied.

During three of the hottest days of the summer Kurt and I worked on the front porch. While he diligently replaced the rotten floor joists, I, in a full Tyvex suit and dust mask, sanded what felt like hundreds of peeling balusters. We listened to a book on tape between exchanging jokes and war stories of terrible jobs we'd had in the past, as sweat poured down my face. Tyvex suits, I learned first hand, become ovens under the hot summer sun.

Dad and I did some dirty jobs together as well. We ripped up ancient carpets, first from the downstairs room that was to be the massage studio, then in the upstairs bedrooms. Dad would attack each one using a utility knife to make the initial cuts. My part came next: with a crowbar in hand I'd start tearing and lifting. It was always a mystery about what lay beneath each old carpet. We always hoped we'd find a beautiful hardwood floor, but that dream never came true. We did find some decent pine floors which we figured we could clean and paint. What we could count on without question was that we would uncover multiple generations of dirt, dead flies, dust, and skin cells.

After a lengthy battle to detach the carpet from one of the upstairs rooms, Dad and I were completely out of breath. We deliberated about the next step and decided to simply throw it out the window rather than carry it down the stairs, through two rooms, and out the back door. Dad squatted at one end of the nasty shag rug; I took the other end; and we rolled it up like an enormous cigar. On the count of three we heaved it out the window. It fell like a canon ball, taking the adjacent gutter down with it. But so what. We'd accomplished our mission of freeing the house from its final wall-to-wall curse. We laughed and exchanged a celebratory high-five. Hell, the gutter was probably already broken like just about everything else in my, by now, beloved old house. Like Frankenstein, it was slowly being brought back to life by our family, and we were the mad scientists in charge of the rebirth.

Downstairs, Dad and I cut a hole through the back wall of the front hallway to accommodate a door that would become the entrance to my massage studio. It was perfectly placed. After entering the front door, clients would have direct access to the massage room with its own little lavatory without impinging on my personal living space. A highlight of the studio was the luxurious cork floor that Dad and I installed together. We had decided that a massage therapist, whose work is conducted primarily on his feet, should have a supportive, cushioned floor. And I appreciate it every day!

Toward the end of the renovation we hired a locally renowned sign maker to create a shingle advertising my new business which I'd decided to call The Blind Masseur. I was so excited to make an appointment with Will Parmalee, a modest and humble genius in my opinion, whose work I had grown up admiring. After I showed him my studio, we strolled onto the front porch which faced High Street. He took a few measurements, pocketed my business card in order to duplicate the logo of two extended hands in red on a sunny yellow background, and said he'd be back with the finished product in a couple of weeks. As he started up his old pickup truck, I couldn't contain the broad smile that spread across the right side of my face. I was going to have a genuine Parmalee-made, neo-Gothic sign promoting The Blind Masseur!

In two month's time, 160 High Street had become not only my home but the location of my new profession—my calling, my life's passion, the fruit of the goal I had worked so hard to attain. In the earlier days of my journey, the days when I could barely rally the will, the desire, or the strength to get out of bed each morning, I could never have predicted or imagined that I could live my life being both blind and happy at the same time. It was my incredible good fortune that I scored the family I got in this lifetime, for they were, and continue to be, pivotal in making this unbelievable dichotomy happen.

I give myself credit, as well, for my conscious decision to live my life to its full potential, facing each obstacle that presents itself with as much courage as I can muster. If this resolve is in any way a gift from a higher spirit, then to that spirit I give thanks and proclaim with confidence, "I'm blind and I'm happy!"

FIFTEEN

THIS PRECIOUS LIFE

This being human is a guest house
Every morning a new arrival.
A joy, a depression, a meanness,
Some momentary awareness comes
As an unexpected visitor.
Welcome and entertain them all!
Be grateful for whoever comes,
because each one has been sent
as a guide from beyond.

~ Rumi

DURING THE YEARS FOLLOWING NEIL'S surgery and blindness, I experienced many of the stages of grief that have been documented and written about by experts in the field of mental health, a prominent voice being that of Elisabeth Kubler-Ross in her 1969 book *On Death and Dying.*

Early on, getting through one day at a time was a monumental challenge for me, and every day that passed I considered a success simply because I had endured it, had put one foot in front of the other, and offered everything I had to support those I loved. Somewhere along the line I discontinued working with my therapist. I convinced myself that I simply didn't have the energy. I couldn't revisit the trauma I had experienced. I had only enough reserve to manage the daily grind of responsibilities and obligations to my job and my family. Talking, processing, analyzing my emotions and state of mind required more inner resources than I felt I had. The very thought exhausted me. I recognize now that I felt alone and isolated from others—not all the time—but I remember that I developed a strongly held belief that nothing and no one could help me. And that was that. That was just the way it was, and I accepted it.

Kubler-Ross maintains that although there is a sequence to the stages of grief, individuals spend different lengths of time working through each step and may express each stage with different levels of intensity. For me, the stage of Shock and Denial lasted a very long time. Of course I knew with every fiber of my being what had happened to Neil. But for a long time, even some years after his hospitalization and treatment, his making his way in the world as a blind person, a weird sensation would happen to me. I'd be driving along or engaged in a mundane household activity, and a wave of disbelief would wash over me, just out of nowhere. And I would say to myself, "I can't believe this happened." As I began to explore this area of my life, I read that shock and denial are defense mechanisms and numbing agents that provide emotional protection from being too overwhelmed.

For me, there was definite overlapping of the stages that Kubler-Ross describes, but I did, at some point, move into the

Pain Stage. According to my reading it can be described in this way: as the shock wears off, it is replaced with the suffering of unbelievable pain. Although excruciating and almost unbearable, it is important that you experience the pain fully and not hide it, avoid it, or escape from it with alcohol or drugs.

None of this literature was in the forefront of my mind or in my radar at all during the experiencing of it, but there was grief movement within me that I was trying to make sense of. The following is an excerpt from my journal from that period:

> *I'm trying to sift through my own thoughts as well as some information I've gathered to understand my meltdown and uncontrollable tears a week and a half ago in my meditation class and continuing through the next morning at home while Jim and I prepared to take our boat out of the water for winter.*
>
> *I seemed to experience a breakdown—or maybe it was a breakthrough—and I was unable to "contain" myself, to hold myself together, to move forward in the everyday manner of living one's life.*
>
> *I found myself in a space, a zone, that I actually had been seeking; a place that I understood I would eventually have to inhabit in order to truly move forward in my life's journey. Whether I could have gotten to this place earlier, with help, I don't know, but a process was surely occurring over a period of time.*
>
> *Four years ago I cried for a period daily. I think the trauma was still lodged in my psyche and my body.*

Disbelief would roll in, unpredictably and often. I guess it is common for disbelief to accompany trauma: you know something has changed forever and is "true." But somehow, somewhere deep inside yourself, it is not yet solid, not firmly fixed, and, therefore, not always "real."

After a period of tears, which happened every day, often with a drink in my hand to take a break from my unfathomable grief, I entered a stage of no tears. During this long stage there was no discharge of grief. It would come rolling in, and I remember thinking and feeling, "This is worse than tears—the pain is so severe." But I would put the pain somewhere. I learned how to bypass it in order to protect myself. I could say, "Not now!" and snap my mind shut to it.

At first when I developed this capability, I didn't understand it. It just became an automatic response. It served me, and it did not serve me to investigate or explore the mechanism of how it worked. But since taking the Transforming the Mind class at the meditation center, it became impossible for me not to question and inquire into how my mind was working.

Most of the reading for the class emphasized that in order to heal from pain, pain must be acknowledged and allowed to run its course, in all its permutations. If evaded or denied, it will follow you, stalk you always. It is impossible to truly move on from it without being brave enough and open enough and wise enough to be present with it.

But I didn't know how to do this. I could read the

words and absorb the message and believe in the truth of it but could not find the door to open and proceed.

However, I understood that the endeavor was an important step for me. I needed to get to this new place. Although I didn't know how, I became open.

I began to see a visual image of what I was doing on a psychological level. I saw a wooden box. And when the pain arose inside me, I stuffed it inside the box, and I packed cotton all around it in all the crevices and cracks and corners. I smothered the pain, and I smacked the lid down on top of it. I stored it away, but that did not mean that it was gone. It still existed in a container that I had created.

Eventually, I must have become primed, ready at last. The focus of the study I was immersed in—achieving peace by transforming the mind—and my willingness to face my pain in order to become free came together that night in class and the holding container started to leak pain. Once started, I could not control or contain it.

At some point during this release of grief, I got it. This was 'being present with the pain,' acknowledging it fully, and absorbing it into my being. I was doing what I had read about but had not been available to do: I was letting go and feeling. This was not happening through my own decision or will; it was happening because I was open to the message, to the advice. The part of me that is intuitive intelligence, not the 'planning' part of me, was freed to step forward.

I wept in the hallway of the meditation center after it was clear I had to remove myself from class; I wept into Judy's arms as she came to comfort me; I wept all the way to Westminster West and as I made my way into bed. I knew something unusual was happening, as I continued my uncontrollable weeping the next morning after rising. I wept getting ready to help Jim remove our boat from the marina.

When Jim questioned my ability to help as planned, I insisted I could. My tears were not debilitating. They were different from anything I had experienced before. It's not that they weren't tears of incredible sadness and anguish—they were. But they were tears of release and acceptance more than defeat and hopelessness.

They were also tears of compassion for myself, for the helplessness I had felt for so long, for my valiant struggle to stay strong in the face of a new existence, a new reality. They were tears for all the love and hope I had mustered and given, for every shred of effort I had put forth when I didn't think it possible to go on. They were tears of praise for my courage and perseverance. These tears were not bitter—they were an acknowledgment of and tribute to all I had endured. They just poured out as I went about the business of my day.

When they finally stopped of their own accord, I felt a calmness. Something had happened to me and within me that was supposed to. I felt that my perspective was broadening. I couldn't expel the grief from my life, but

it no longer had the power to completely dominate me. I could recognize it, face it, co-exist with it.

~

Following this experience I reflected upon my resilience to life's low blows. I couldn't pretend that I wouldn't still grieve each time a new limitation in Neil's life reopened the channel of sorrow within him. But would I be somewhat stronger, quicker to recover? I felt that I might be, although I wasn't sure. I wondered if experience had made me any more equipped to deal with future sorrows, the inevitable ones that await all of us who are connected by virtue of our human birth. Again, I did not know. In the end, I had to make peace with the possibility that being human means we cannot help meeting our losses and pain as beginners, always.

~

One weekend, I drove out to the showroom of blacksmith Ian Eddy whose work I admired. Our house had a few items I'd purchased there years before, a wrought iron paper towel holder and several wrought iron toilet paper holders, and I wanted to buy some more.

Years ago, I had met Ian and his wife Jenny when we attended the same birthing group: Jim and I were expecting Jessica, and they were expecting their son. Although our paths had rarely crossed over the years, I still had fond memories of that counter-culture group of young adults who'd come to Vermont to raise their young families.

As I entered the shop, I was greeted warmly by Jenny. I told her that I was on a mission to duplicate the same items that Jim and I had enjoyed for so many years. As she rang up my purchases, she asked me how I was.

I had not intended to say anything to Jenny about Neil; I found it too overwhelming, too inappropriate to bring up the trauma we'd endured in a casual encounter. But as I looked at Jenny, I knew she knew. I said, "I don't know if you heard that our family had gone through some hard times a few years back. Neil was diagnosed with a brain tumor and the result of everything is that now he is blind."

"Yes," she said, "we had heard. Tell me, how is he doing?"

"He's doing well," I reported.

Then out of my mouth came a statement I'd never uttered before, had never even formulated in my thoughts until that moment: "There's nothing—nothing—that can keep Neil from living his life."

"Good," she said. And her face softened, relaxed. "I'm so glad to hear that."

And there it was, suddenly before me: a revelation, a conviction. We human beings are hard wired for survival. At almost all cost we wish to live, to participate, to contribute, to be included, to be recognized and valued for who we are and what we bring to the world. I witnessed this resolve almost daily in my son; I'd also learned the truth of it through my obsessive reading about the suffering of others who managed to lead fulfilling, meaningful lives against all odds. The memoirs and accounts that had sustained me, given me hope, all seemed to point to the same truth.

Andrew Solomon in his book *Far from the Tree* interviewed dozens of families who lived with the stress of parenting children with a variety of disabilities. He found that after a period of shock upon realizing that the life they got was not the life they'd envisioned came a time of psychic reorganization. And following that, most people, after a few years, returned to the level of happiness at which they'd lived prior to the dramatic event that changed their lives.

I know for a fact that Neil would tell you in the same afternoon that being blind is an absolute nightmare and that he is a happy guy. The paradox is hard to grasp. But the mystical aspects of existence often are.

∾

A handful of times during Neil's living in his downtown apartment and then at 160 High Street, I'd phone him in the evening and say, "Hey, I don't have to be up and out tomorrow morning as usual. Let's have breakfast together at your place. Make an extra cup of coffee for me. I'll bring eggs and English muffins."

"Great!" he'd answer. "See you when you get here!"

I'd arrive, make myself at home in his kitchen, and then, sipping coffee at his kitchen table, we'd chat.

For me, mornings hold promise. The day is young and

fresh and full of potential. It may, in the end, turn out to be humdrum or disappointing, but in the morning, you can't know that. In the morning it is possible that the upcoming day will hold a success or reveal a happy surprise. For Neil, however, mornings also brought forth feelings of nostalgia.

"It's so great to have you here," he told me on more than one of our shared mornings. "This is sometimes one of the loneliest times of day for me. I get up by myself and make coffee just for me. I wish I had someone to experience it all with— the beginning of a day, the plans, the feeling of togetherness. I have so much love to give. I wish I had someone to share it with."

"Neil," I would say, "I wish it too, with all my heart," feeling my chest contract with the all too familiar pain of yearning for things to be different. "And I think that it's entirely possible that it could happen some day. You're a wonderful person, and I know you have so much to offer."

Soon after, we'd hug good-bye, each of us heading into our own day. And I would feel sad. But, over time, my sadness for the things that felt cosmically denied to Neil did, indeed, cut me less deeply. I'd come to terms with the fact that I could not fix everything that brought us sorrow. While I could listen with compassion and assure Neil that his pain was more than reasonable, my being overcome and incapacitated with grief didn't help him, and it was damaging to me. This understanding did not emerge as an "Ah-ha" moment of sudden illumination. I did not make a conscious decision to change my outlook and my behavior. I think I quietly, over time, became worn down from the swings between relative stability and intense, agitated emotion. My body, my being, my self could no longer endure it.

But there was more. Neil no longer appeared fragile and at-risk to me. He had endured so much, had grown in so many ways, had come so far. He was living not the life he'd imagined but the life he got, with strength and dignity and resolve. I could be sad for Neil without grasping so desperately for the things that might never be. Of course I wished deeply for him to have love in his life. What parent doesn't want that for his or her child? But if that never happened, he would survive. There would be a hole, always, but despite the inevitable holes, he could, and would, carry on. I had developed faith that Neil had what it took to forge a life worth living.

∼

In December 2013, just five years shy of Neil's original diagnosis, he suffered a set-back. Over the years we'd become accustomed to continued good news following his brain MRIs. Neil had graduated from a schedule of brain scans every three months to every six months. It had felt like such a positive step and an affirmation that all would be well in the months and years ahead. I had become so confident in his sustained good health that I no longer required Jim to be with us as we waited for Dr. Renaud to review the latest pictures shortly after Neil's emergence from the MRI canister. I had come to expect, to count on, Dr.

Renaud's usual bustle into the exam room, computer under his arm, with the announcement: "It looks good!"

He would then, as always, show us the images taken just an hour earlier. The comparisons had held steady over the years: stability in the area of the original tumor with no regrowth. Buoyed by the good news, relieved of the undertones of anxiety, we had many merry times in that little exam room. And Neil would always phone Jim from the car on the way home before reclining his seat in order to shut his eyes for half an hour. While the trips to University-North offered great happiness in the knowledge that we did not have to think about the next one for a good long time, they were exhausting for both of us.

"Oh, no!" I proclaimed upon opening the December appointment notice from the hospital. "What are the chances! Neil's MRI appointment is scheduled for the day I have my own doctor's appointment. I'm just going to have to cancel mine and reschedule for a later date."

"No, Alison," Jim interjected. "Keep your appointment. It's been on the calendar for weeks. I'll take Neil. It's not a problem for me. I don't have anything else I have to do that day."

"Well, it may not be a problem for you, but it is for me," I countered. "It's too difficult for me not to be there when Dr. Renaud comes in with his report. I would go crazy being anywhere else. I know me, and I would be biting my nails and pacing the floor from wherever I was."

"Don't be silly," answered Jim. "Everything will be fine."

Neil spoke up from his perch in the kitchen where he was finishing lunch following a work-out and hot tub with his dad.

"Mom, keep your appointment. Let dad take me. I promise to call you from the car on the way home."

"OK," I agreed. "I know the routine. Just don't forget to call."

~

The call never came. I began to feel anxious as the approximate time I expected to hear from Neil came and went. I went over and over his schedule in my mind: when his MRI was set to begin; the amount of time I knew it took for the procedure to be completed; the hour it took for Dr. Renaud to receive the images; Neil's time in the neurological oncology waiting room; his time sitting in the exam room waiting for Dr. Renaud. All of this should have happened. They should be driving home by now. Why had Neil not called?

The idea of calling Neil's cell phone, of course, entered my mind. But I was on the highway, driving back to Westminster West from my own appointment. I knew I couldn't handle bad news at such a time. I was in no way prepared, and my instincts sent out a warning signal to keep going, to keep calm, to stop imagining the worst. I began to conjure all the possible scenarios for a logical delay in Neil's day: the nurses had more than their usual trouble inserting the IV line into Neil's deeply embedded and seemingly narrow veins, and the special IV team was not immediately available; Dr. Renaud had been paged for an emergency; Jim and Neil had had car trouble on the way up. I didn't believe any of these, but I hoped beyond hope that Jim's car would not be in our driveway when I arrived home so that an unforeseen scenario was, indeed, the logical explanation.

But the car was parked in our driveway as I knew it would be. I ran into the house, yelling, "Jim, tell me what happened at Neil's appointment! What was the reason I never heard a word! Where are you? Where is Neil?"

Jim appeared at the top of the stairs and began to descend toward me. "Neil is at home where I dropped him off after the appointment. We didn't call you because we didn't want to upset you. Things didn't go as well today as they had at other appointments."

I felt light-headed, disoriented, literally, beside myself.

"Of course I'm upset; I've been upset for hours. I knew something bad must have happened. Tell me everything!"

We moved to the living room where I balanced uneasily on the edge of the couch, and Jim continued.

"Dr. Renaud came in as usual and said, 'Everything looks good.' He brought up the original tumor site on the computer while Neil let out a whoop and we high-fived. I looked at the scan, like always, comparing it to earlier ones when all of a sudden Dr. Renaud got quiet and said, 'Oh, no, there's something potentially troubling in another area of the brain.' He immediately got on the phone to Radiology, and they discussed the image. It appears that whatever it is—it's more in the area of the brain stem— is not taking up blood, which is good. So it's not acting like a tumor. But he's concerned about it, and he wants Neil to come back in two months rather than six. It could be nothing, or it could be the beginning of another tumor."

"Oh my God," I retorted. "I cannot believe this is happening after all this time! I feel sick. Tell me—how is Neil doing?"

"He's upset, of course. We both were. We were flying high one minute and completely deflated the next. But we went to McDonalds for lunch, and I think I cheered him up. I got him laughing. Of course, he's concerned about you."

I called Neil immediately. "Neil, I just heard about your day. It must have been awful. I'm so sorry you had to go through this. But it could be nothing. Remember one time, early on, we got a call from the oncology office saying something on the MRI looked problematic? And it wasn't. The next time you had an MRI everything was fine. I'm choosing to think that will be the case this time. It happened to us once before, and that's what's going to keep me steady for the next two months."

"Mom, it was a total bummer. I just couldn't believe it. I was actually doing a little jig before the bomb fell. But I'm OK."

He sounded tired and resigned to the turn of events that the day had delivered—that he was going to have to live with "not knowing" for a period of time.

"There's nothing I can do about it, so I'm just going to carry on as usual," he said.

"Well, that's what I'm going to do too, Neil. That's our

plan. And I feel better. We'll be OK."

"I'm counting on it," he said as we hung up.

But already our life had changed.

*n*FOR NEARLY FIVE YEARS MY BRAIN MRIs were fine, and we got used to living on solid ground. My family and I were elated when after several years of regular good news Dr. Renaud changed my MRI schedule from every three months to every six. Happily, there had never been evidence of regrowth at the tumor site, a possibility that would need to be monitored regularly. I had absolutely no reason to think that anything would change. I was in top form and felt strong and healthy and positive about my future. I had built, and was continuing to build, a good life.

While I can't say we were nonchalant when MRI days rolled around, we were, on the whole, pretty relaxed about them. Usually Mom and I made the trip together and called Dad on the way home to fill him in. It was always great to feel we could put our next visit completely out of our minds for half a year. We'd feel high all the way down Route 91 South.

In December 2012, just a month shy of the five year anniversary of discovering the malignancy that had invaded my brain, Dad and I made the pilgrimage to University-North together. My mother must have had some important obligation that kept her from accompanying us. I know we must have convinced her that all would be well, as usual, and assured her that we would give her a call from the road.

Following the MRI and lunch, Dad and I headed to Oncology. After a short wait in one of the private exam rooms, Dr. Renaud came in and told us that things looked stable as usual, and I knew he was bringing the image up on the computer screen for my father to look at.

"No change to the remnants of scar tissue at the tumor site," he said.

Dad and I performed our well-practiced high-five followed by our usual celebratory remarks—then stopped short as Dr.Renaud's voice changed suddenly from bright and light-hearted to concerned and serious.

"Wait a minute...." I heard.

He had apparently scanned away from the image of the original tumor site to an area where there had been no trouble in the past and now saw a peculiar growth, small but definitely new, and troubling. My father and I were shocked into silence in the face of this startling new reality. Time just folded in on me though I was aware that Dad began asking Dr. Renaud about his opinion and possible next steps to determining what it might be. But I was somewhere else, beyond details and the ability to focus. My mind was a cascade of confusion, though the one thought that surfaced and seemed to solidify was this: after everything I had gone through, six weeks of radiation, a year of chemotherapy, and all the "in-between" stuff, I thought I'd had it beat. And now I had to endure the news that there might be an entirely new tumor.

Dr. Renaud felt that the best plan was to wait two months, repeat the MRI, and check the area again for signs of growth or shrinkage or change in general.. Although I thought it was a good sign that he was not freaking out about it on the spot, it meant that I would have to live in "wait and see" mode for a stretch and make my peace with that.

Dad and I endured a long, heavy-hearted drive back home. Despite his optimistic, encouraging words— "Neil, we've overcome far more than this, and we don't know for sure if it's even a tumor at all"—there was no denying that we were both upset. And we knew that one of the hardest parts still before us was sharing the scary news with my mother who was anxiously awaiting what we'd all expected to be a call of relief and cheer. But this just wasn't a call we could make from the car.

TRUE TO OUR COMMITMENT, WE did carry on as usual during our two month wait. Aside from Jessica and Jackson, we told no one of the thunder cloud we lived beneath. Neil immersed himself in his massage practice; Jim and I spent February in Florida; and Neil flew down to spend four days. We didn't speak of our anxieties as there simply was no point. We would show up at University-North at the appointed time on the appointed day and go from there.

In mid-March, I sat in the waiting room of Radiology waiting for Jim and Neil to emerge from the changing room where Neil was dressing after his MRI. We'd grab some lunch in the cafeteria before heading to meet with Dr. Renaud in an hour's time. As I sat with my magazine, I glanced sideways and saw Dr Renaud walk briskly past the front desk and disappear into the inner sanctums of the Radiology Department. I knew instinctively why he'd come. He wanted to view Neil's scan immediately rather than wait for it to be sent to his office. He probably wanted to confer about it in person—review it thoroughly before seeing us. There was surely nothing foreboding in seeing him here. But somehow it did serve to ratchet my nervousness to an even higher level.

～

The news wasn't what we wanted to hear. The unexpected growth had enlarged a bit over the past eight weeks and was now taking up a tiny amount of blood. It was definitely a small tumor. It was located in an area of the brain that could potentially affect Neil's balance, and Dr. Renaud asked Neil whether or not he was experiencing any such symptoms. Neil told him he had no symptoms. He went on to pass the neurological exam with his usual flying colors. He was in fine form and feeling as strong and healthy as ever. Neil and I quietly held hands, and I laid my head on his shoulder. I think, for a moment, we all observed the disappointment and sadness of the situation, the dashed hopes that we would never again have to live through this particular nightmare. And then Jim moved us into the next moment: "So what are our options? What are the treatment plans that lie ahead?"

Dr. Renaud told us that he had already spoken to Dr.

Carrington, Neil's neurological surgeon from five years before. In fact, he had made an appointment for Neil to see Dr. Carrington the following week. They had conferred and agreed on two points, that surgery was not an option due to the risks of permanent loss of balance; and a biopsy must be done to identify the type of tumor, thereby informing treatment options. The big treatment unknown was this: whether it was possible or advisable for Neil to undergo another round of radiation, a plan which would never be considered if regrowth had occurred at the original tumor site. Dr. Renaud planned to confer with Neil's radiologist at Southside Medical Center. Things were moving faster this time. There would be no suspension in Limbo for round number two.

The biopsy revealed that Neil's stage-two tumor was the same type as the original tumor. Given that Temodar had proved effective at the original site, a course of twelve cycles of the drug became the game plan. The thorny decision regarding another round of radiation took the longest. The upshot was that after much conferring with colleagues in Boston, Neil's radiologist in southern New Hampshire informed Dr. Renaud that in Neil's case a second course of radiation was deemed a positive element in his treatment.

I felt glad that careful consideration had gone into weighing possible risks versus benefits and hoped that the addition of the radiation to the chemotherapy would provide the power needed to eradicate this small but threatening tumor. I also thought how ironic it was that, in the end, Neil would have a second crack at keeping his white Darth Vader radiation mask as a keepsake. Because this time, he'd be bringing it home to his house, not mine.

~

"Neil, I've heard great things about you," smiled Dr. Carrington as he grasped Neil's outstretched hand. He was still slender and youthful-seeming after five years. "You're an inspiration to all of us, and I want to tell you, this could be just a bump in the road for you."

I looked at this man who'd been a major player at the start of this journey and recognized that as kind, as sensitive, as openly friendly as he was, I was counting on never having to see him in a professional capacity again. But here we were. And, despite the circumstances, my heart filled with gratitude for the special gift of his encouraging words. They touched me deeply, offering the hope and resolve I so desperately needed to move into this next challenge. More than once during the second full year of Neil's treatment I'd pull out Dr. Carrington's gift. I'd put my arms around my strong, brave son and say, "Remember, Neil, this is likely just a bump in the road for you."

THE BIOPSY, CONFIRMING A SMALL, stage two malignancy, thrust me into old times. Once again I would have to slog my way through another round of radiation and twelve cycles of oral chemotherapy. But just as a sequel to a blockbuster movie can never rival the original, this ordeal became just one more hurdle in life, a few steps back in my journey of healing, and mundane in comparison to the first episode. It was a major drag, and I certainly won't downplay the gravity of the situation, but, as we had already proved to ourselves, my family and I, there is nothing we can't handle together. And that's what we staunchly set out to do.

*a*FOLLOWING NEIL'S SECOND DIAGNOSIS, I found myself sinking once more into a vortex of disbelief and despair. And I ask myself now whether this sinkhole was the same one that held me for so long years earlier or whether it was different, a new make and model. The shock of Neil's original cancer diagnosis, his blindness, his formidable challenges, both physical and emotional, had been so unexpected, so unfamiliar, so extreme, it sucked our family into a new reality. But the new reality was not new any longer. And we had endured, matured, and gained the kind of life experience we would have done anything to avoid.

Nevertheless, I cried anew following Neil's set-back and felt separate from my fellow human beings. I felt that as hard as we had tried to keep our chins up, to rebuild our lives, to accept, with gratitude, Neil's different life, we were marked for continued sorrows. More than anything, I couldn't bear to tell our family and friends. Not only did the saying of it inflame my fear of the future, but I hated adding worry and sadness to the lives of people I loved. Their hearts would carry a new heaviness due to their love and concern for us. Telling was a hard task. It was for me, and I know it was for Jim and Neil as well.

In addition to plummeting into sorrow, I was pulled, once again, into the abyss of bewilderment. But it was somewhat different this time in that I could recognize it, name it, and remember it. Because I had emerged from my first bewilderment with a commitment to facing the truth of how things are, including the nature of how our minds and the Universe work, I was able to question the stories I had woven over the years to sustain myself. Had I truly believed that a set-back was not in the realm of possibility for Neil? Or had I so strongly "willed" it not to happen that belief got a toe hold in my mind and pushed its way to center stage? I had to confront the possibility that I had constructed a world of magical thinking.

What is magical thinking, and how does it happen? Is it universal or only constructed by the neediest of us? Is it ever helpful? And what happens when it is exposed for what it is—a crutch, a "blankie," a lie? What then? What are we left with to shepherd us through the hardest parts of our lives?

Some time ago I read about happiness in Sharon Salzberg's best selling book *Lovingkindness: The Revolutionary Art of Happiness*. She explained that the common tendency of human beings to feel some bitterness in the face of another's good fortune or happiness is based on a misconception. We tend to feel that there is a certain set amount of happiness in the Universe to go around. If our friend or neighbor is fortunate, the happiness supply is lowered a bit; there will be less to spread around and, in all probability, not enough left for us. Sharon exposes this magical thinking as contrary to the way the Universe actually works. There is not a fixed or static amount of good fortune in life. There is no bottom, no end to happiness and good fortune.

In a different, but similar vein, I realized that I held the child-like belief (or maybe just hope, based on a wishful illusion of justice) that a person who had suffered greatly had paid his or her dues. It seemed to me that in a just and orderly world, suffering SHOULD be a limited commodity. In my mind, Neil had withstood more than his fair share of pain. He had accepted it, endured it. And now it must be someone else's turn. That would be the fair thing. Bad luck should be divvied evenly, spread around equally.

When I write it now, it seems laughable, ridiculous. Yet I know I'm not alone in my naïve, delusional thinking. Elisabeth Kubler-Ross contends that "bargaining" is a natural reaction to feelings of helplessness, vulnerability, and a lack of control that is hard to make peace with. I recognized that I had, indeed, woven stories to sustain me, to comfort me, to provide me with hope and a measure of peace. I had convinced myself that unconditional love and support are enough to boost the immune system, that exercise and healthy living are guaranteed, protective benefits, that being a good sport, keeping to the sunny side, not complaining or blaming, somehow earn cosmic merit.

The return of Neil's cancer had cracked the cocoon I sheltered in, the cocoon of my own making. With my refuge in shards, there was no choice but to emerge, still and always me, but with my eyes no longer averted, looking out instead at the truth of how things are: that life is hard and precious at the same time; that fear, sorrow, despair, and anger can exist side by side with joy, hope and love; that the anxiety of "not knowing" is tempered by the joy of experiencing the mysteries that life holds; that the power of love can transform us into bigger, more courageous versions of ourselves than we ever could have imagined.

Neil completed his second full year of treatment with relative ease. He was stronger and healthier this time around. He was able to keep up his business, his exercise regime, his travel and speaking schedules. And he met Katy, the love of his life and life partner. In true Neil style, he ended the year with a second chemo-free party—this time in his own home with seventy well-wishers.

Through no choice of my own, for me, the past eight years have been a wisdom journey. There were times along the way when I was proud of the person I was becoming and times I felt estranged from myself. And I would have to say that that holds true today. Sometimes I am strong; sometimes I am weak. Sometimes I remember the important lessons and truths, and sometimes I don't. Often joy washes over me, and just as often, fear or despair set in. I am all of these emotions and states of being, and none of them all the time. And there is comfort and freedom in the knowing of that.

Jim and I were given a little boy to nurture and raise

alongside his brother and sister. We couldn't have known when we held him for the first time that sorrow was lurking or how entwined our three lives would, of necessity, become. Since the day of the call that changed everything, we have scaled the cliffs of hope and slid into chasms of despair, hanging onto each other every step of the way. We opened our eyes—those that could see and those that couldn't—to the many blessings that life had set aside for us. We gained some vision we might not have been privy to had our lives been easier. And we gave thanks along the way, and do to this day, for the life we got.

SIXTEEN

PEAKS AND VALLEYS

Life isn't about finding yourself.
Life is about creating yourself.

~ George Bernard Shaw

*A*S OFTEN AS I TOLD MYSELF that I was living a good life—I could do what I wanted, eat when, where, and what I chose, wash my dishes when I needed to use them again, make my bed or not, answer to no one but myself—I knew there was an undeniable void in my life. Although I appreciated being surrounded by loved ones, at the end of every day they would return to their homes and their own lives. I had had five years of practice becoming comfortable living by myself. And as much as I was proud of my self-reliance, I never really became accustomed to being alone.

It wasn't easy for me waking up each morning to endless darkness, forcing myself to get out of bed and methodically making my way to the kitchen to get the coffee going. I would turn my little radio on to Morning Edition, not because I was dying to hear what was going on in the world but rather to have the company of someone else's voice as I sipped my coffee in solitude. It was equally painful at the end of each day. As I brushed my teeth, I'd wish I had someone who really cared about, and benefited from, my careful oral hygiene. Then I'd slip into my cold, lonely, too-large bed, waiting for my own body heat to warm it up. Often, I'd lie awake, yearning for the solace of sleep to stop my mind from wandering into sorrowful places. I was still a young man with so much love to offer, yet no one seemed interested in acquiring a free ticket.

I was almost resigned to the idea that I might never meet my soulmate, someone I would joyfully share the rest of my life with. I certainly didn't want to become a bitter old hermit, the stereotypical old guy who yells at little children to get the hell off his lawn! In truth, however, beyond these occasional self-demeaning thoughts and images, I was so glad to still be here. I recognized in myself an inner determination to keep moving on with my life, with immense gratitude to be alive after all that had transpired. Even so, much of the time I was lonely.

On an evening when I was feeling tired and not particularly social, I had to grapple with the fact that I'd been invited to a neighbor's birthday party, had agreed to attend, and now just wanted out. I was on the verge of calling my ride to say I was feeling under the weather, but I decided I would go after all. I mean what was I going to miss—another Saturday night alone at home listening to another book on tape? Besides, I had made a pledge to myself a while back to accept social invitations, to get out and do things, even if the prospect seemed challenging. Little did I know that this decision would turn out to be the best one I ever made.

Shortly after my driving acquaintance and I arrived at the celebration, I ended up on the couch, an all too familiar party venue for me. As usual, I tried to look relaxed and happy, a bit nervously tapping my leg to the beat of the music coming from the next room, my half smile indicating I was open for party-type banter. During the next fifteen minutes I responded with exuberance to three greetings from voices I didn't recognize and whose owners neglected to identify themselves. In short order, I regretted my decision to come. I missed the serenity and comfort of my own home, yet, as usual, I had no means to act on my change of heart. So I sat, pretending to take pleasure in the background music while contemplating when I could reasonably ask for a ride home.

Immersed in planning mode, I barely felt the cushion on my left side compress as someone sat down beside me. Before I had a chance to begin my customary greeting, I felt my couch companion move in closer so I could hear her voice over the music and general party cacophony. She introduced herself as Katy, taking my hand to shake it in a formal introduction. She told me that she'd come over to join me because I looked lonely taking up the whole couch by myself. I laughed awkwardly, saying, "All the more room for me to rock out to the music," at the same time, admitting inwardly, "If you only knew how right you are!" We conversed for a while in an easy natural manner before she excused herself to use the bathroom. As she got up, she added, with a totally winning little giggle, that I should save her seat because she wasn't done with me! I teased her back, saying I would protect her seat with my life. She laughed again, leaving me alone on the couch which now felt too empty and too big. As promised, she quickly returned and asked if I wanted to go out on the porch as it was a lovely, warm evening, and we could get some fresh air. "Fresh air sounds good," I agreed, rising from the couch that I had assumed would be my assigned spot for the entire evening. But now she was leading me effortlessly through a small crowd of people and out onto the porch where we found two plastic chairs and pulled them close together. We spent the rest of the night conversing on the porch and were barely bothered by the smoking crowd who could have cared less about fresh air!

Katy told me that we were, in fact, neighbors, as she lived a mere six houses west of me. She had seen me on the sidewalks of High Street and had noted The Blind Masseur sign hanging from my front porch. As we conversed, I learned a bit about her life. She had been raised Catholic, but she quickly became disenchanted and rejected her religion at a young age after discovering she could not become an altar girl. After high school she attended Wesleyan College for two years, then dropped out to travel around the country with friends. She and her high school sweetheart had a baby together at the tender age of twenty-one. After they separated, she raised her daughter on her own with the help of her parents in order to finish college. She raised her child much the way I had been raised—eating organic food, no TV, a simple country lifestyle. Along the way she had become a certified public accountant in order to provide for herself and her daughter.

As we moved on to exchanging tales of foreign travel

and outdoor adventures, our mutual excitement grew. We had so much in common! One topic led to the next, and time just flew by. How could this evening have shifted so quickly from counting down the minutes until I could leave, to experiencing it move way too fast? Most women I'd conversed with—women I might have shown a slight interest in—would soon run out of things to say, leaving us both with long embarrassing silences as we struggled to rekindle the conversation. I'd come to recognize the challenges that others feel in conversing with a blind person. I had witnessed this new reality with people I used to chat with freely and easily. But with Katy everything was different. Our conversation that evening flowed as effortlessly as water. It was an equal exchange. Neither one of us monopolized the conversation or fell into uncomfortable silence. By spending the entire evening with me, this girl named Katy went well off the beaten path where other women trod. I was overcome with how unique she was. I knew then and there that I had just met the woman I'd been waiting for. Her obvious kindness and generosity—her very outlook on life—left me infatuated and wanting more of her company. But, unbeknownst to me, my ride had been searching for me and now was more than ready to go. So, without trading numbers, Katy and I parted ways. I walked away from the most divine moments I'd shared with a female companion in over five long years.

That night I was unable to fall asleep or to stop thinking about the evening I'd just spent. However, as I lay in my bed, the pessimist in me took control. I doubted that I would see Katy or, more literally, hear from her again. Consequently, I told myself, it would be best to let go of the memory of our short time together— deliberately put it behind me— as it probably meant nothing to her other than showing sympathy for a lonely blind guy. A week later, however, Katy showed her genuine interest by calling to see if I'd like to get together. I was overjoyed!

Much later in our relationship, Katy shared with me that a month before we met she had drawn up a list of things she wanted to do, accomplishments she hoped to achieve, challenges she promised to undertake in order to enrich her life. One of the items on her list was definitely intimidating and something she had never done before. That item was to ask someone out on a date! As we laughed together about her confession, it struck me that of all the potential candidates she could have asked, she chose me. And that made me the luckiest man in the world!

In response to Katy's call to "get together," I invited her to my house for morning coffee. It was the best I could come up with. She arrived with a home-made peach pie, and while we had a fabulous time just being in each other's company, Katy still teases me that rather than being wined and dined at a fancy restaurant, it was the tamest first date of all time! I totally agree, but, in my defense, after five rusty years, I was out of practice and needed to go slowly. In any case, after our first, low-key date, we quickly became inseparable. I began caning my way up to her front door (about one hundred sixty-seven steps, give or take a few) and marveled at the luck of it all that the woman I was enthusiastically courting was so accessible!

∾

At the time Katy and I met, I was taking heavy duty chemotherapy to battle the second tumor that had brought us all up short. So, on a double take, I was not exactly holding a winning hand. But she proved, once again, to be the woman who ventured out where no one else had dared tread. One evening, during my five days "on" cycle, I made the mistake of downing my poison pills and turning in for the night without taking the accompanying, necessary (I learned) anti-nausea drug. I became violently ill during the night, throwing up the entire contents of my stomach including the chemo pills. When there was nothing left to expel, I spun into an endless cycle of dry heaving. Retching without the benefit of expulsion is one of the most painful and exhausting involuntary acts the body sometimes succumbs to. Not being able to sleep, and finding myself in a somewhat altered state, I decided to e-mail Katy at two in the morning to tell her about my pathetic mishap, using a bit of humor to offset my misery.

Instead of being turned off by my condition, Katy showed up at six A.M. before leaving for work, letting herself in with the key I had given her, and found me curled up tightly, sweat-soaked and shivering in my bed. Despite the lingering aroma of vomit and without concern for her professional clothing, she lay beside me, gently stroking my head and telling me she wished she had been there for me during those agonizing hours. I was overwhelmed with gratitude for her presence but relieved that she hadn't witnessed my nighttime state-of-being. Despite her soothing effect on me,

I couldn't help but feel low. Here I was, deathly ill and helpless in front of a woman I wanted to impress enough that she wanted to be with me. But I realized later that this was not, in fact, a low. I had chosen not to hide the state I was in. And the result was that I got to witness Katy's bravery, and I got to fall deeply in love with her and the beautiful spirit she embodied.

After about a year and a half and hundreds of trips back and forth to each other's dwellings, we made the decision to move in together. Katy put her place up for rent and moved in with me at 160 High Street. I couldn't have been happier on the day we moved her last truckload of belongings into what was now our house. I had turned thirty-five years old. Katy was the first woman I had ever lived with, and she was totally worth the wait!

∾

Soon after we met, Katy followed a lead that reintroduced the thrill she knew had been torn from my life. Many mornings on her way to work she listened to a podcast called Dirtbag Diaries which features outdoor activities all across the world. On this particular morning the organization being discussed grabbed her attention immediately, and she began to feel excited. It was called Paradox Sports, and its mission was to enable those with disabilities to get out into the wilderness and learn to climb rock and ice.

For the past three years, since hearing that podcast and following up on an organization that had "me" written all over it, Katy and I have been intimately involved with Paradox Sports. We have rock climbed at The Gunks in New York so many times that certain routes have become familiar to us. Every winter since we began our relationship, we have ice climbed with Paradox at the Cathedral Ledge in North Conway, New Hampshire. And, of course, we have met wonderful new friends. Although she was an avid hiker, Katy had never climbed before, but true to the woman she is, she was game for anything! Due to her natural athleticism and love of adventure, she excelled at it from the start. She is supremely happy one hundred feet off the ground with crampons dug into a frozen waterfall and perfectly driven ice axes holding her securely, with only her blind boyfriend on belay.

~

With Katy by my side, or perhaps I should say "ahead of me," I am happy to report that my experience with tandem biking did not end as I was pretty sure it had. It, like me, took on a new and unexpected life.

One of my father's favorite co-workers, Maria, offered me her husband's beautiful tandem that had been gathering dust in their garage. The frame was high quality, but it was not suited for the more demanding off-road trails that Katy and I dreamed of using it on. At the same time I received this generous gift, my sister's good friend Angela and her husband Dan and family moved to Brattleboro. To say the least, Dan is a bike aficionado. He owns thirty bikes which he's collected over the years. He and I took the new tandem out on a test ride and realized that it needed a lot of work to become what I wanted. Dan took the tandem home with him along with my two bikes which I had cherished in my sighted days. He removed a number of specialty parts from my own bikes—all the hard-core mountain bike components— and transferred them onto the tandem. In the end, we created something amazing. Our design plan and his mechanical know-how transformed the once tame bike into the gnarliest tandem imaginable! My beloved Katy and I are thrilled to be riding our tandem, which we lovingly call "Brutus," on terrain we couldn't have covered using the original bike, as beautiful as it was. I love the fact that it, like me, had two distinct lives. We regularly ride on the West River trail, and each time I have the pleasure of reliving what mountain biking is all about. It makes me feel athletic again. Katy commands the controls, the shifting, the braking, and I am the heavy peddler—the bike's outboard motor—which Katy appreciates. We are bonded by our love of exercise and of being outdoors for the benefit of both our bodies and our spirits. And we are both grateful for this special gift that came our way.

∼

Last year, Katy and I planned and saved for a trip to Colombia, South America. Every evening for several months before this highly anticipated adventure, we sat together on our living room couch studying Spanish. Although our preparation was making me as excited as she was, I became aware, at some point, that we needed to face some potentially hard facts. Because I can tell Katy anything, I had to share with her my nervousness that this ambitious trip might take a toll on our relationship. For me, given my blindness and limitations, a foreign environment—once a thrill for me—was now an undeniable source of fear. This would be my first experience post-blindness in a distant country, amid new people, an unfamiliar culture, speaking a foreign language. In many instances I would have no idea what was going on around me. I was concerned that my unique situation, with its unavoidable dependency on Katy, would result in her possible resentment towards me. Our upcoming trip might prove more difficult than anything we had yet experienced, and I might try her patience at times. I joked that I might occasionally feel like a heavy, cumbersome piece of luggage she was forced to drag behind her everywhere we went. Katy chuckled at the image but did not dismiss the seriousness of my doubts.

Because of our love for each other and the trust that had grown in the light of that love, I chose not to internalize these worries, letting them fester until they grew out of control. I openly expressed my fears as I had been learning to since the beginning of our shared life. As we lay in bed I told Katy how grateful I was for the amazing patience she'd displayed throughout our time as a couple. In a soft voice, she told me that she understood, as well as she could, the vulnerability I felt. In the next breath she assured me that we were a team—we were in this together—and that she relied on me as her faithful male companion whose build, alone, would scare off any potential ne'er-do-wells, and she playfully squeezed my bicep. We both broke into laughter. But a huge, burdensome weight that I could not bear alone was lifted from my shoulders.

And, happily, our time in Colombia was an unforgettable adventure for both of us. The worries that had competed with my eagerness to travel, that had worn away at me, did not pan out as I had dreaded. To the contrary, our traveling together was seamless. Neither of us ever raised a voice to the other in frustration. For anyone, disabled or not, feelings of vulnerability can unexpectedly creep up when traveling in unfamiliar territory. And many times you have only your partner to rely on which can be a heavy load to bear. But this trip proved to be a highlight of our relationship and brought us closer together than anything we had encountered so far. For me, it stands as further testament to Katy's courage and uniqueness of being, not only in choosing to live life with a blind partner but in understanding and accepting that adventure always involves some challenge—and that it's totally worth it.

~

While Colombia was beyond successful, another trip required an immediate change of plans while we were far from home and tested our partnership in a completely different way. In the middle of winter 2015, we flew to Colorado to climb with Paradox Sports and then to visit a close friend who'd grown up in Vermont. From Colorado we were due to fly to Longboat Key, Florida, to visit my parents. Mid-trip, while we were still in Colorado, Katy got word that her father was succumbing to the cancer he had lived with for the past few years. We dropped everything and got a direct flight to Charlotte, North Carolina, in order for Katy to spend the last few hours by his side.

The few hours turned into ten long days of nearly full-time living in the hospital, monitoring her dad's daily, then hourly, status. And we did it together. Minutes after his death I held Katy's grief-stricken body against me, and I could actually feel her pain entering my own body. I tightened my hold on her, trying to absorb more of the pain. I wanted to provide some ease from the newness of her loss. Trying to imagine what she felt in those moments, my mind went to the unthinkable, the unbearable: what it would be like to lose my own father. And I knew, without a doubt, that Katy would be right there to hold me during my own time of suffering, as I was for her.

∼

Best of all, for me, are the simple comings and goings of household life with my partner, my soulmate, my girl. Katy and I love to cook together. She has most certainly broadened the horizons of my rather limited diet which consisted of countless veggie burgers, bowl after bowl of cereal, be it for breakfast or dinner, and my classic favorite— microwave tuna melts. Katy is now the resident Martha Stewart, and I am her loyal sous chef. I am responsible for crafting a creative salad while she works happily at the stove where sounds of vegetables simmering or salmon sauteing are music to my ears. We take pleasure in inviting friends or family for dinner. We pull the kitchen table away from the wall, extend the leaf, converse and laugh, and delight in one of Katy's signature delicacies. Under her tutelage I have grown leaps and bounds as a cook myself. I've become accustomed to procuring a filet of the finest Faroe Island salmon from our local co-op while Katy is at work. By the time she walks through the door, the fish will be wrapped in foil with a sinful amount of melted butter and baking at three fifty. My days of relishing frozen pizza above all other meals are happily in the past.

~

During our earliest days of getting to know each other, I discovered that Katy and I had a similar sense of humor regarding life with all its joys and all its sorrows. And it quickly forged a tight bond between us. Whether listening to an outlandish stand-up comedian or cringing together at the blatantly insensitive remarks of a bully politician, we were of one mind regarding the often ludicrous nature of life. There are no easy answers to fall back on, so why not just rejoice in the craziness of it all, recognize that we are not in control, throw up our hands in a response of joy and submission, and go along for the ride? Together!

Of course, my extended family fell head over heels for Katy as quickly as I did. They could see that she made me comfortable in my own skin. In her orb, I lost the sinking sensation of inadequacy that had been stalking me for years, the feeling that I had somehow failed in life or come up short in my efforts to adjust. She only knew me as blind, and that was the person she fell in love with. Her habit of treating me as an equal is so life-affirming that it makes me feel reborn. When we walk together, she describes everything I am missing with seemingly no added effort and without a hint of sympathy in her voice. She never overhelps me, opens the car door for me, shows me directly into the men's room, or backs me into a chair in a restaurant. In turn, falling in love with Katy was the most effortless thing I have ever done!

At home or abroad, I am a lucky man. I am blessed to be loved by the most uplifting person I will ever meet. Though I can't literally see it, the smile that graces her adorable face is intoxicating to me and always contagious.

~

I admit that I'd always been on the fence as to whether or not I wanted a guide dog in my life. I often felt that I barely had the ability to take care of myself, let alone another living being. Did I want to routinely take a large dog outside to go potty? Did I have the energy or motivation to take it on more than one walk each day? Did I have faith enough to put my life at possible risk by "blindly" following behind a dog? I wasn't absolutely sure I could rally the love and constant attention that was expected of me. To sum it up, was I ready for the commitment that owning a guide dog would entail?

Even in the face of my doubts and concerns, however, it was hard to resist the enthusiasm that Katy and some of my family members expressed on the subject. Those in favor believed that a guide dog would vastly broaden my horizons. High on the list of pluses they cited were greater independence and loyal, round-the-clock companionship that would enrich my life. Eventually I became convinced. I contacted a guide dog school here in New England and began the application process. I was well aware that there were differences and, therefore, options regarding guide dog schools sprinkled throughout the northeastern United States. My decision to apply to the New England school was based on two factors: first and foremost, it raises and trains only German Shepherds. The school's commitment to Shepherds appealed to me as there is, in my mind, a certain powerful, noble, even regal quality inherent in the breed. Having done a bit of research, I learned that German Shepherds are one of the most intelligent breeds and that their loyalty to their owners is unsurpassed. And, secondly, unlike other schools that run residential programs on their own campuses, the New England school believes that training in your own environment is preferable. The school sends a trainer to your home, your neighborhood, your town for two weeks. This made greater sense in my life as I did not want to leave my massage therapy practice, my work-out practice, or Katy. And I was sold on the idea of my dog becoming immediately familiar with my stomping grounds with our instructor by our side.

I awaited a response to my application which I assumed would come via e-mail, text message, or a simple phone call. To my surprise, my acceptance arrived via regular mail. One day, Katy came across the letter from the New England school amid a pile of junk mail and a couple of bills lying on the floor beside the front door where the mailman had slipped it through the mail slot. We joked about an organization for the blind sending a written communication but didn't linger on it. Nothing could dampen our excitement about the new member of the family who was about to join us! According to the letter, each dog is carefully chosen to best match the profile of each recipient, and because of that, it might be two months time before my dog and trainer would show up on my doorstep.

So the wheels were turning! Another new endeavor—another leap into the unknown—was about to begin for me. I did not dwell on the possibility that this new venture would not be successful. Yes, I had known faculty at The Carroll Center who had not had positive experiences with guide dogs. And I tried to ignore a red flag in my own circle of acquaintances.

During my first full year of treatment, when I was living with my parents in Westminster West, my friend Rich and his wife adopted a German Shepherd that had failed out of the same guide dog school that I had committed to. Of course I had many questions about why his new dog, seemingly gentle and sweet, had not met the necessary standards to work as a guide, but the organization had not shared that information with Rich. It was simply not necessary now that this dog was deemed best suited as a household pet. Twice a week I had taken slow, leisurely walks with Rich and his now beloved pet down the quiet rural road that ran through Westminster West village. This was early in my recovery, so I was not yet a vigorous walking partner. I remember being arm-in-arm with Rich as the dog, on his leash, walked calmly in front of us. From time to time, Rich even had me take hold of the leash. I remember thinking that maybe someday I would be able to make this same walk alone with my own loyal guide dog.

∼

In the end, only a month passed before I received a telephone call from my soon-to-be instructor, Michael. He informed me that he'd be making the trip to Brattleboro in two weeks with my very own dog and that we'd begin our training the day after my dog and I made our acquaintance. He sounded like a great guy from our brief conversation, and I felt confident that we'd get along well and enjoy working together. Of course, I wanted to know everything he could tell me about the dog: what sex it was, what its name was. I hoped it wasn't something ridiculous like Bingo or Chandler. But for some reason Michael could not share that information on the phone. He told me I'd learn everything in two weeks time.

By now, it was early December, maybe not the best time of year to start on this new venture given the harsh Vermont winter that lay ahead, but I sat out on my deck the morning of Michael's arrival, bundled up in multiple layers and feeling very excited. Right on schedule I heard a vehicle pull into my driveway, the tires crackling a thin sheet of ice that had formed the night before. I heard the door open and close as I made my way to the edge of the deck and stood at attention waiting for Michael to make his way over to me. He greeted me with a pleasant voice and a powerful handshake, and I welcomed him to my home. I was surprised he didn't have my dog in hand as I'd expected, but he said that the dog was waiting in the car. Our first step was a brief orientation without the dog being a front-and-center distraction for me.

I led him inside to my living room couch and prepared to listen closely to the information he was about to cover. Before beginning, however, he told me what I was dying to know: my dog was a male and his name was Zen. Michael probably sensed my excitement as I repeated the name softly a few times,"Zen, Zen"—I had already fallen in love with it! I was quickly brought back to the business at hand when I felt Michael place something onto my lap. This, he said, was Zen's working harness, the leather harness with the short, square handle Zen would wear whenever we were out together. We covered a few more essential items on his checklist, and then Michael announced that the time had come to meet Zen. Before he brought him into his new home, however, Michael asked me to close a couple of the interior doors so that Zen could concentrate on me without the distraction of having an expanse of new environment to explore.

I closed off the door to the upstairs and the back room, and Michael went out to get him. I was filled with a kind of heightened energy, and I paced through the kitchen and living room rather than try to contain it. I even, ridiculously, pondered what posture or position I wanted to be in when Zen saw me for the first time. I heard them climb onto the deck, and I went to stand in the living room so Zen would see me as soon as he turned the corner from the doorway. As Michael led him through the kitchen, I heard his doggy nails clicking across the linoleum floor in his eagerness to greet me. Michael warned that Zen was a bit overexcited to be in a new place and to meet a new person, and, true to his words, Zen jumped up on me before Michael could pull sharply on his leash. To show that Zen's exuberance did not alarm me at all, I got down on the rug and began petting him vigorously and making formal introductions.

He was absolutely gorgeous, I could tell. I nuzzled up against his strong neck, and I loved his smell. As I hugged him with both arms, I felt we would be the closest of friends for life. He responded to my physical affection by licking my face in between pulling on the leash that Michael was firmly gripping. I didn't even take note of his rambunctiousness. Why wouldn't he be brimming with energy and curiosity under the circumstances?

Michael wanted to know if I was comfortable with Zen staying overnight after meeting him for the first time. I responded quickly that, without question, Zen would stay with me from this day on. Michael laughed, sharing that some people feel a bit overwhelmed at the first meeting with their future guide dogs and are not quite ready to take on immediate responsibility for them, and that's understandable and totally OK. I assured Michael that not only was I ready for Zen, but I was so excited and honored to work with the two of them, and I looked forward to the next two weeks. As he handed me Zen's leash, Michael said he was just as honored to work with me and was looking forward to tomorrow, our first official day. I appreciated his kind words, of course, but as I shook his hand good-bye, I knew that no one could be as grateful and happy as I was on this day.

~

The following morning Michael emphasized that the first critical step in the training regimen is creating a strong bond between owner and guide dog. There can be no shortcuts in the process: it takes time, effort, and commitment, and it can feel somewhat isolating, as many days must be devoted almost exclusively to the development of this relationship. No one but I was to greet or interact with Zen. He needed to learn that I was his sole provider. Only I could ever offer him food or the doggie treats that would be used in his training. And Michael emphasized that Zen had never, and never should, sample human food. He was a service dog, a working dog, who should be ignorant of table scraps so he would never be guilty of the inexcusable act of begging.

While this prescribed first phase of our life together intrigued me—this conscious building of his loyalty to me and only me—I felt, at the same time, that my wings had been clipped. It was lonely staying at home seeing no one but Michael each day for our training sessions. When Katy arrived home from work she would avert her eyes from Zen and stay clear of where he was tethered to the couch as he learned to adapt to his new home and surroundings.

As time went on, however, Zen and I were able to branch out. We routinely had play times in the house. I would throw his ball from the living room all the way into the kitchen, and he would barrel after it at full speed. I could hear his legs skidding to a screeching stop as he caught up to the ball and grabbed it between his teeth. We began going to my parents' house so I could renew my workout schedule with my father and have lunch with my mother. My parents were now able to greet Zen, pat his lovely head, and acknowledge his existence. But he seemed excitable. When people ventured near him when he was off-harness, off-duty, he would jump up on them just like any young, untrained dog. He was young and energetic, to be sure, and I knew I had to give him what he needed in that department—enough exercise for his age and temperament—but "untrained" he should not be. This just didn't seem right to any of us, but try as I did to correct this unexpected bad habit, he was not able to calm down and change his behavior. Over Christmas time with my extended family all gathered at my grandmother's farm, Zen's obviously unruly behavior caused me embarrassment and angst.

My family began, one at a time, to show up for training sessions with Zen, Michael, and me. Concerned about what they were seeing and listening to my frustrated reports that one day would seem to go well, causing me to feel encouraged and positive, but the next would feel like two steps back, they decided to trail behind us and learn what they could in an effort to help me. They were becoming increasingly anxious about my official training period being a mere two weeks. My mother was particularly concerned about two sections of one of our routine routes. On an outing with us, she noted that Zen did well leading me around trash cans and sign posts, but two of the roads we needed to cross to make our way downtown were small but busy one-way streets. And neither had a traditional curb. The curbs were no different from all the driveways we passed along the way. I would try to anticipate when we were nearing one of these roads and give my command, "Zen, find the curb," to alert him to stop. Fifty percent of the time he did stop. But fifty percent of the time he'd just venture out, and Michael would grab me back and have the two of us practice it again. At one time or another both of my parents asked Michael if he thought Zen would settle down and become a reliable, trusted, first-rate guide dog. He said that, yes, he thought so.

But a red flag went up for me when Michael was forced to change Zen's collar three times during the first few days of training together. Zen always started out well during training sessions but soon seemed to lose his concentration and become distracted by too many things—squirrels scampering, birds flying low, other pedestrians, random scents he picked up along the sidewalk. And god help us if we passed another dog on a leash. I couldn't predict if and when Zen would veer from his job of keeping me safe, as he regularly deviated from staying on track. It didn't take Michael long after following behind us to assess that the traditional collar was not doing the job. He instructed me to jerk up on the leash in order to give the collar a quick, attention-getting tug and to command, "Leave it, Zen!" in a deep, authoritative voice. Once it became clear that I was doing exactly as he instructed, he substituted the traditional collar for a gentle leader. This collar is designed to go around a dog's snout so that when the leash is pulled, the dog's nose is lifted, preventing it from sniffing the ground. It is meant to insure that the dog stays in proper form. The gentle leader did, at first, seem to do its job, but, in the end, it wasn't enough to keep Zen on task.

It seemed apparent that nothing gentle would do the trick. So we moved to a toggle collar. Made of metal, it tightens around a dog's neck when the leash is jerked upward and is designed to snap a dog back into compliance. Zen barely seemed to notice it. Finally, we graduated to a pinch collar, and the name doesn't really do it justice. Simply feeling it made me grimace. It is a metal collar laced with about a dozen metal spikes and resembles a barbaric torture device. It works by digging into a dog's throat when any tension is applied to the leash. When I shared my reaction with Michael, he assured me it was a temporary measure to get Zen on the right track. I silently wondered why Zen had been sent to me with a lightweight, traditional collar when it had so obviously been the wrong choice for him. And why had Michael not known this in advance?

By the end of the official training period Zen was still doing a spotty job of guiding me around Brattleboro. I could not count on him maintaining continual focus and keeping me from bumping into a sign, a potted plant, or some outdoor seating. My bruised shins were evidence of these mishaps. After two and a half weeks of training, Michael informed me that we had completed the curriculum, and I was now at the point where I would be working with Zen on my own. If I had any questions or concerns I should call the school, and a trainer could be sent right away to check in on us. I tried to think positively about moving on to this next step, but I couldn't help picturing Michael throwing up his arms in resignation as he abandoned me and this questionable guide dog he'd been assigned to work with. As his vehicle pulled out of my driveway for the last time, was he breathing a sigh of relief that this futile assignment was behind him at last?

∼

One of our first solo walks, a simple stroll Zen and I had practiced with Michael regularly, was a straight shot down High Street with a curve to the right onto Main Street where we were to meet my friend Laura. But it went awry, partly my fault for not "feeling" my way to the right as I should have but partly Zen's for subjecting me to a potentially dangerous situation. Before long, I suspected we were off course because we had been walking for much longer than usual. Just as that sinking, humiliating sensation of knowing that we were off track began to set in, a concerned pedestrian called out, "Do you know that you are in the middle of the street?"

Apparently Zen and I had turned in the wrong direction on Main Street, and at some point he had veered from the sidewalk and proceeded up the middle of the busiest street in town. A long parade of traffic had formed behind us, too polite, baffled, and apprehensive to lay on their horns at an obviously blind man following his adorable yet misguided guide dog.

I quickly sidestepped to the left until I hit the curb and tripped my way back onto the sidewalk. Swallowing my humiliation, I thanked the kind gentleman profusely as he led me back in the direction where Laura sat in her wheelchair waiting and wondering where I could be. She certainly was surprised to see me being led by a stranger from the opposite direction she expected. Before my rescuer transferred me to her custody, he kindly but pointedly advised her to "keep an eye on this guy!" This cringing mishap undermined my confidence in going out alone with Zen, so I continued to practice with family members and my ever-helpful, ever-willing, ever-optimistic friend, Rich, who came by once a week to practice with Zen and me.

On harness, in public places, Zen was easier and better-behaved. In restaurants, in hospitals, he would tuck himself quietly at my feet under a table or chair. He was so quiet and content that it was not always evident that he was there. When he was noticed, we received many compliments from passers-by regarding his beauty and his behavior. But these settings concealed his unresolved behavior issues.

∾

After several months of living together, Zen and I had an established routine around meal time. I would measure out the proper amount of dry food and fill the bowl with water so that it would soften as I'd been instructed to do. Ten minutes later his food would be the right consistency, and I'd put the bowl on the floor in his designated eating corner and let him roam free in the kitchen to eat his meal.

I had told Katy as she was leaving for work that morning not to worry about dinner. I would have it prepared by the time she got home from work. Earlier in the day Zen and I accompanied my mother to the supermarket, and I had picked up one of those perfectly cooked, meat-practically-falling-off-the-bone rotisserie chickens. Now that dinner time was fast approaching, I got busy preparing a salad before Katy arrived. I sliced up a pepper, some cucumber, baby carrots, and a perfectly ripe avocado, and added them to a base of fresh spinach. I could practically see the bright colors of my delectable creation. "Five-star restaurant," I told myself as I pushed the salad bowl to the back of the counter so I wouldn't inadvertently knock it onto the floor with a careless sweep of my arm. Now it was time to prepare the main course. OK, maybe it had already been prepared by someone else, but Katy wouldn't dwell on that, and isn't the presentation half the game? I removed the chicken from its container, pleased that it was still warm. I began to strip the tender bird of all its meat, placing each piece carefully on a large plate which I then stacked on top of the salad bowl at the back of the counter. I felt proud of my domestic abilities. I had just prepared a meal fit for my queen with a little help from Stop and Shop. I was blind, but I didn't need to wait for my girlfriend to come home after a long day at work and prepare a meal. I checked my audible watch. It was five fifteen, perfect timing, as Katy was due to arrive at five thirty. I had just enough time to clean up and set the table. I shuffled over to the sink to give my greasy hands a proper wash. When I was through, I'm not sure why, maybe to stroke my ego one more time, I checked our meal. I ran my hands cautiously across the counter so as not to knock the plate of chicken off the salad bowl. I located the salad bowl and followed it up to the plate which was wet but empty. I guessed that I hadn't oriented myself correctly. I lifted the plate up and felt that, indeed, it was sitting atop the salad. As I ran my hand across the counter in front of the bowl I felt and then picked up a single scrap of chicken. I was shocked! Suddenly my mind put all the pieces together, yet I still couldn't believe what had happened. During the few minutes I had taken to wash my hands, Zen had jumped up and placed his front paws on the counter, and leaning as far forward as he could, he had eaten the entire chicken I had placed at the very back for safekeeping!

I didn't know how to react; no words came to mind. How could he have done this? It was the ultimate betrayal! While I had had the water running so I couldn't hear him, Zen had jumped up and gorged himself on my fine dinner. This was something even a bad dog would never do let alone a fully trained guide dog. Zen had supposedly been trained to be an irreplaceable aid to me, to work with me not against me. My mind went to dark, irrational places. It felt as though Zen knew I was blind, and he took advantage of it. For the first time I really wanted to spank the shit out of him, but I did not and never would. I think he knew he had done wrong as he was hard to locate. Once I got my hands on him, I chastised him the only way I knew how—"Bad boy! Very bad boy!" And I led him to his tether on the wooden couch leg. I returned to the kitchen utterly crestfallen and reexamined what I already knew was a total loss. I threw the now empty plate into the sink and went over to the corner to confirm what I already knew I would find. The meal I'd set out for Zen was wholly untouched.

～

The winter that Zen came into my life was a record-breaker for snowfall in the northeast. But every morning I got out of bed at six o'clock to usher him outside for his morning trip to the loo, a.k.a. my back yard. My audible outdoor thermometer informed me that it was nineteen degrees as I climbed into my felt-lined boots and zipped up my parka. I had Zen on his gentle leader as we slowly made our way down the slippery ramp attached to the back deck. I maintained a wide stance with my knees slightly bent, taking baby steps as we descended to the driveway which was particularly icy this morning. We were about halfway to the back yard when my feet suddenly slipped out from under me, and I came crashing down on my right hip. The impact caused my hand to release its grip on Zen's leash, and in a flash, before I could recover and reach for the dropped leash, he was gone. I staggered to my feet and called him to come back to me as I limped into the back yard. Part of me could not believe that Zen would abandon me in my time of need, lying on the frozen ground, dazed and in pain after a fall. I would have thought he'd stay by my side, my pain being his pain, licking my face and whimpering for me to get up. Another part of me, however—the more realistic side, less prone to whimsical fairy tales about the unbreakable connection between man and his faithful dog—knew, from his previous behavior, that my well-being was not even on his radar.

After yelling out his name to no avail, it soon became clear that Zen had no intention of coming, and I knew I hadn't a prayer of finding him, so I changed direction and pointed my bruised body back to the house. All sorts of thoughts were swirling through my mind as I located the ramp and entered my back door, most of them in the form of potential headlines in the local newspaper: "Man loses forty thousand dollar guide dog," or "Two year old guide dog is killed after being hit by a car on High Street."

Luckily Katy was still home. I frantically yelled upstairs for her to come down and help me as Zen had gotten away! She had just emerged from the shower, but she threw something on, raced downstairs and out the door in pursuit of him. She located him in what felt like the longest two minutes of my life. She led him back, reporting that he was exploring the neighbor's back yard, nose to the ground, oblivious to any drama that had happened in his own back yard. As Katy handed me the leash, I thanked her with all my heart for coming to the rescue and did my best to hide my shame for the mess I had made of a seemingly simple morning routine. But she totally picked up on my feelings of frustration and failure as she always does. She put her arms around me and pulled me close, assuring me that everything was OK and that we would always have each other's backs. I lay my head on her shoulder soaking up the calmness that Katy invariably provides for me. In her arms a feeling of well-being returned, even with my hip throbbing and Zen pulling on the leash.

Nevertheless, I phoned the guide dog school as I'd been instructed to do if I felt the need for extra support or another trainer's perspective on the troublesome behavioral issues that Zen continued to display. They immediately consented to send someone up for an assessment. I was to get Zen into his working harness, and the new trainer and I would walk a familiar route and confer about his observations.

On the day of his arrival I waited on the deck with Zen half suited up, his pinch collar on, and his harness beside us. As the man got out of his vehicle and walked up the ramp onto the porch, Zen did what he always did when a visitor approached: he spazzed out. When the man reached the top of the ramp, Zen lurched at him, stopped only by my strong grip on his leash which I had choked way up on in anticipation of his standard behavior. As the fellow came closer, greeting Zen by name with what I recognized as a well-practiced, calm, yet authoritative voice, it made no difference. Zen started jumping up on him as I worked to keep him in control. The assessor asked me if this was typical behavior, and as I continued to suppress Zen, gritting my teeth in effort, I assured him that this is what I dealt with every day. He asked me to hand him the leash which I gladly did. After three or four minutes of working with Zen, attempting to get him to calm down, yanking on the leash, and calling out the commands that were part of Zen's training repertoire, he got no further than I had. And then he came out and said what I'd been waiting the last three months to hear: "This behavior is totally unacceptable!"

As soon as I heard those words—not from my father, not from a friend, not even from an objective observer, but straight from the mouth of an expert sent from the very training school which had sent Zen to me—well, I cannot articulate the feelings of complete relief that washed over me. For so long I believed it was my fault alone that resulted in our troubling failures.

The assessor walked Zen down the ramp and put him in the back seat of his vehicle then returned to the deck to speak further with me. I asked him questions: "Is what you observed normal behavior for a two year old newly trained guide dog? What could I have done better?" His responses were, "Absolutely no" and

"Nothing that I could see." He asked me if Zen was showing any signs of improvement, and I had to answer honestly that on the well-practiced walk downtown, even after all this time, I couldn't rely on him stopping at two important intersections. He had put my life in danger more than once, and, as a result, I could not trust his guidance. The assessor replied, "That is all I need to hear. I am going to take him back with me."

We never even took a walk with Zen. The assessor had made the decision there and then that this situation was untenable. All he'd had to do was walk onto my deck, approach my guide dog, and ask me several pertinent questions.

I gave him everything that belonged to Zen: his enormous bag of food, his treats, his extra leashes and assortment of collars, his chew toys, his various fetch balls, even the soft, luxurious bed I'd purchased for him. I wanted to sever every connection with Zen. I didn't want my hand to brush across his old leash as I was reaching for my jacket, reminding me of this tumultuous and failed experience.

I listened to the assessor's vehicle pull out of my driveway just as I had months earlier when Michael departed, only this time Zen was leaving rather than staying. The assessor had mentioned something about the possibility of Zen being retrained and returned to me, but I knew that would never happen. In my mind, Zen was not destined to be a guide dog, and I would not see him again. We had spent five long months together, yet I was happy to have him go. It felt strange to me, but I knew I would never regret my decision to give him up, and I felt the deepest sense of release. I felt twenty pounds lighter as I entered my house and closed the door behind me and behind this era of my life. And I recognized two emotions simultaneously: sadness and freedom.

I walked slowly up to my bedroom and into my closet where I located my abandoned white cane. I dusted it off before bringing it downstairs and putting it in its old place by the back door. And I thought of Zen as I made this conscious switch, of his undeniable beauty, of his strong physical form and adorable floppy ears, of his playfulness and skill at intercepting a ball in mid-air. And I wished him well in whatever new life awaited him.

I've learned over the course of the past eight years that there is a silver lining to most any situation, and there is one that emerged from my time with Zen. After our training and practice on the route from busy High Street to downtown, I lost much of my fear of traffic that had held me back in my independent mobility efforts. After Zen's departure, I decided to up my efforts with my cane. I realized that I had become so familiar with this particular route that I had committed it to memory. I now feel confident in my ability to cane my way to Main Street where Laura waits for me on our usual corner.

∼

Today I can say that I am more than content: I am happy—a statement I wouldn't have believed ever proclaiming at the outset of this ordeal. Facing the prospect of death at a young age propelled me into gratitude for each day I live and for every one I'd be granted down the line. I can't help but feel gratitude to that higher spirit for the breath I draw into my lungs, for the sun's warmth on my skin, for the joy of hearing the voices of my loved ones, for the subtle scents of one season giving way to the next. While sadness casts its shadow over me and probably will as long as I live, as that is the nature of shadows and sadness is a given in all of our lives, I have much to celebrate. I have love in my life, physical endeavors that challenge me, a calling that inspires me, a successful business in a vibrant town. I have witnessed through the living of my life these past eight years, as well as through the reliving of it in writing this memoir, how fragile yet how resilient we human beings are. I feel privileged for the miracle of that awareness and hope that this memoir stands as a testament to it. We are all here temporarily, whether that is at the forefront of our minds at any given moment or not. I have viewed this project, this memoir written together with my mother, as a token of my time here. I hope those who read it take heart in its message that despite overwhelming odds—a devastating loss and what will likely be lifelong limitations—I wake up every morning still here in this crazy, beautiful world, knowing that each day is one more gift.

ACKNOWLEDGMENTS

Love and gratitude beyond measure for our reader, editor, and dear friend, Judy Coven. Her insights and inspirations, her meticulous attention to detail, and her unwavering dedication to helping get this book launched into the world kept us moving forward with determination and excitement.

Thanks to Maureen Moore for shepherding us through the self publishing process and especially for the many thoughtful suggestions on ways to shape a book written by two separate individuals. We recognize the patience it takes to work with beginners!